Entzündungshemmende Ernährung

Genießen Sie Wohlbefinden und Energie mit naturbelassener, entzündungshemmender Küche - Einfach und gesund leben

I0467096

Bathilda Koch

Inhaltsverzeichnis

Einführung in das Buch

Herzlich willkommen zu Ihrem neuen Begleiter auf dem Weg zu einem gesünderen und erfüllteren Leben. Dieses Buch, Entzündungshemmende Ernährung: Genießen Sie Wohlbefinden und Energie mit naturbelassener, entzündungshemmender Küche - Einfach und gesund leben, ist das Resultat jahrelanger Forschung, Leidenschaft und praktischer Erfahrung. Es soll Ihnen nicht nur Wissen vermitteln, sondern Sie auch inspirieren und befähigen, Ihre Ernährungsgewohnheiten nachhaltig zu verändern.

Unsere moderne Lebensweise hat uns oft von der Natur und von traditionellen Ernährungsweisen entfernt. Die Folgen sind weitreichend: Viele Menschen leiden unter chronischen Entzündungen, die zu zahlreichen gesundheitlichen Problemen führen können. In diesem Buch erfahren Sie, wie Sie durch eine bewusste und gezielte Auswahl an Lebensmitteln Entzündungen bekämpfen und Ihr Wohlbefinden erheblich steigern können.

Dieses Werk gliedert sich in mehrere Kapitel, die jeweils verschiedene Aspekte der entzündungshemmenden Ernährung beleuchten. Im ersten Kapitel legen wir die Grundlagen und bieten eine Einführung in die Prinzipien dieser Ernährungsweise. Wir beleuchten die wissenschaftlichen Hintergründe und erklären, warum bestimmte Lebensmittel entzündungshemmende Eigenschaften besitzen. Hier erfahren Sie, welche gesundheitlichen Vorteile Sie erwarten können, wenn Sie diese Ernährungsweise in Ihren Alltag integrieren.

Im zweiten Kapitel widmen wir uns den Lebensmitteln und Nährstoffen, die eine zentrale Rolle in der entzündungshemmenden Ernährung spielen. Sie lernen die wichtigsten Zutaten kennen und erfahren, wie sie auf den Körper wirken. Dieses Wissen ermöglicht es Ihnen, bewusste und fundierte Entscheidungen zu treffen, wenn Sie Ihre Mahlzeiten planen und zubereiten.

Die folgenden Kapitel bieten eine Vielzahl von Rezepten, die speziell entwickelt wurden, um Ihre Ernährung abwechslungsreich und schmackhaft zu gestalten. Von Frühstücksideen, die Ihnen einen nährstoffreichen Start in den Tag ermöglichen, über energiereiche Mittagsgerichte bis hin zu entspannenden Abendessen - jede Mahlzeit ist darauf ausgelegt, Ihre Gesundheit zu fördern und gleichzeitig den Gaumen zu verwöhnen. Sie finden hier auch köstliche Desserts und gesunde Snacks, die frei von entzündungsfördernden Zutaten sind.

Ein besonderes Highlight dieses Buches ist der 30-Tage-Essensplan, der Ihnen hilft, die Theorie in die Praxis umzusetzen. Dieser Plan bietet Ihnen eine klare Struktur und erleichtert den Einstieg in die entzündungshemmende Ernährung. Ergänzt wird der Plan durch eine detaillierte Einkaufsliste, die sicherstellt, dass Sie stets alle notwendigen Zutaten zur Hand haben.

Warum ist dieses Buch anders als andere Ernährungsratgeber? Es verbindet wissenschaftliche Erkenntnisse mit praktischen Ratschlägen und einer Vielzahl von leckeren Rezepten. Es ist nicht nur ein Leitfaden, sondern auch eine Inspirationsquelle, die Ihnen zeigt, dass gesunde Ernährung weder kompliziert noch langweilig sein muss. Die Rezepte sind einfach nachzukochen und erfordern keine exotischen Zutaten. Sie sind so konzipiert, dass sie leicht in den Alltag integriert werden können, unabhängig davon, wie viel Zeit Sie zur Verfügung haben oder wie erfahren Sie in der Küche sind.

Darüber hinaus legt dieses Buch großen Wert auf Authentizität und Menschlichkeit. Es soll nicht nur informieren, sondern auch motivieren und begleiten. Die Texte sind in einem zugänglichen, freundlichen Ton verfasst, der Sie ermutigt, neue Dinge auszuprobieren und Veränderungen mit Freude anzugehen. Sie werden feststellen, dass gesunde Ernährung viel mit Entdecken und Genießen zu tun hat.

Kapitel 1: Grundlagen der antientzündlichen Ernährung

Einführung in die antientzündliche Ernährung

Entzündungen sind natürliche Reaktionen des Immunsystems auf Verletzungen oder Infektionen. Sie sind zunächst einmal ein Schutzmechanismus des Körpers, der uns hilft, schädliche Einflüsse abzuwehren und Heilungsprozesse einzuleiten. Wenn jedoch Entzündungen chronisch werden, können sie zu einer Vielzahl von gesundheitlichen Problemen führen, darunter Herzkrankheiten, Diabetes, Arthritis und sogar bestimmte Krebsarten. Chronische Entzündungen sind oft das Ergebnis einer ungesunden Lebensweise, die durch falsche Ernährung, Stress, Bewegungsmangel und Umweltgifte begünstigt wird.

Eine antientzündliche Ernährung zielt darauf ab, diese schädlichen Entzündungen zu minimieren. Sie beruht auf dem Verzehr von Lebensmitteln, die entzündungshemmende Eigenschaften besitzen, und auf der Vermeidung solcher, die Entzündungen fördern. Diese Ernährungsweise ist reich an Antioxidantien, Omega-3-Fettsäuren, Ballaststoffen und sekundären Pflanzenstoffen, die alle eine schützende und heilende Wirkung auf den Körper haben.

Ein wesentlicher Bestandteil dieses Ernährungsstils ist die Betonung auf natürliche, unverarbeitete Lebensmittel. Obst und Gemüse stehen im Mittelpunkt dieser Ernährungsweise, da sie reich an Vitaminen, Mineralstoffen und Antioxidantien sind, die freie Radikale bekämpfen und Entzündungen reduzieren können. Besonders Beeren, Blattgemüse, Kreuzblütler wie Brokkoli und Kohlsorten sowie farbenfrohe Gemüsesorten wie Paprika und Karotten sind hervorragende Beispiele für entzündungshemmende Nahrungsmittel.

Vollkornprodukte spielen ebenfalls eine wichtige Rolle. Im Gegensatz zu raffinierten Getreiden enthalten sie alle essenziellen Nährstoffe und Ballaststoffe, die zur Aufrechterhaltung eines gesunden Verdauungssystems beitragen und Entzündungen im Körper reduzieren können. Haferflocken, Quinoa, brauner Reis und Vollkornbrot sind nahrhafte Optionen, die in Ihre tägliche Ernährung integriert werden sollten.

Eine weitere wichtige Komponente dieser Ernährungsweise sind gesunde Fette. Ungesättigte Fettsäuren, die in Nüssen, Samen, Avocados und fettem Fisch wie Lachs, Makrele und Sardinen vorkommen, haben nachweislich entzündungshemmende Wirkungen. Insbesondere Omega-3-Fettsäuren, die reichlich in Fischöl und Leinsamen enthalten sind, können die Produktion von entzündungsfördernden Molekülen im Körper hemmen und somit chronische Entzündungen reduzieren.

Neben diesen Hauptbestandteilen sollten auch Hülsenfrüchte wie Bohnen, Linsen und Erbsen regelmäßig auf dem Speiseplan stehen. Sie sind nicht nur hervorragende Proteinquellen, sondern auch reich an Ballaststoffen, die zur Reduktion von Entzündungen und zur Förderung einer gesunden Darmflora beitragen.

Dieser Ernährungsansatz legt zudem großen Wert auf die Verwendung von Gewürzen und Kräutern, die natürliche entzündungshemmende Eigenschaften besitzen. Kurkuma, Ingwer, Knoblauch und Zimt sind nur einige Beispiele für Gewürze, die in der Lage sind, entzündliche Prozesse im Körper zu modulieren und gleichzeitig den Speisen einen köstlichen Geschmack zu verleihen.

Es ist auch wichtig zu verstehen, welche Lebensmittel gemieden werden sollten. Verarbeitete Lebensmittel, die reich an Zucker, Transfetten und raffinierten Kohlenhydraten sind, können Entzündungen fördern und sollten daher gemieden werden. Ebenso sollten Sie den Konsum von rotem Fleisch und verarbeiteten Fleischprodukten einschränken, da diese häufig gesättigte Fette und entzündungsfördernde Stoffe enthalten.

Die Umstellung auf diesen Ernährungsstil erfordert möglicherweise einige Veränderungen in Ihren Essgewohnheiten, aber die Vorteile, die Sie daraus ziehen können, sind immens. Es geht darum, bewusstere Entscheidungen zu treffen und eine tiefere Verbindung zu den Lebensmitteln herzustellen, die Sie konsumieren. Dabei ist es wichtig, geduldig mit sich selbst zu sein und die Umstellung Schritt für Schritt anzugehen.

Ein praktisches Beispiel für den Beginn Ihrer Reise zur entzündungshemmenden Ernährung könnte darin bestehen, Ihren Tag mit einem nährstoffreichen Frühstück zu beginnen. Ein Smoothie aus Beeren, Spinat, Leinsamen und einer pflanzlichen Milchalternative ist nicht nur lecker, sondern auch vollgepackt mit entzündungshemmenden Nährstoffen. Zum Mittagessen könnten Sie einen Salat aus Blattgemüse, Quinoa, Avocado und einem Dressing aus Olivenöl und Zitronensaft genießen. Das Abendessen könnte aus gegrilltem Lachs mit gedünstetem Brokkoli und Süßkartoffeln bestehen. Diese Mahlzeiten sind Beispiele dafür, wie einfach und schmackhaft diese Ernährungsweise sein kann.

Kapitel 2: Lebensmittel und Nährstoffe, die Entzündungen bekämpfen

Die wichtigsten Bestandteile der entzündungshemmenden Ernährung

Um Entzündungen im Körper effektiv zu bekämpfen, ist es von entscheidender Bedeutung, bestimmte Nahrungsmittel und Nährstoffe in die tägliche Ernährung zu integrieren. Diese Bestandteile zeichnen sich durch ihre entzündungshemmenden Eigenschaften aus und tragen wesentlich zur Verbesserung des allgemeinen Gesundheitszustandes bei.

Beginnen wir mit den Früchten und Gemüsesorten, die eine herausragende Rolle in der entzündungshemmenden Ernährung spielen. Beeren wie Blaubeeren, Erdbeeren und Himbeeren sind reich an Antioxidantien und Polyphenolen, die helfen, freie Radikale zu neutralisieren und Entzündungen zu verringern. Insbesondere die Anthocyane in diesen Beeren haben starke entzündungshemmende Effekte. Darüber hinaus sind Zitrusfrüchte wie Orangen, Zitronen und Grapefruits vollgepackt mit Vitamin C, einem weiteren kraftvollen Antioxidans, das die Immunfunktion stärkt und entzündliche Prozesse im Körper reduziert.

Grünes Blattgemüse, darunter Spinat, Grünkohl und Mangold, sollte ebenfalls regelmäßig auf dem Speiseplan stehen. Diese Gemüsesorten sind reich an Vitaminen, Mineralstoffen und sekundären Pflanzenstoffen, die entzündungshemmend wirken. Der hohe Gehalt an Vitamin K in grünem Blattgemüse unterstützt die Regulierung der Entzündungsreaktionen und trägt zur Knochengesundheit bei.

Kreuzblütlergemüse wie Brokkoli, Rosenkohl und Blumenkohl enthalten Sulforaphan, eine Verbindung, die nachweislich entzündungshemmende und krebsbekämpfende Eigenschaften besitzt. Regelmäßiger Konsum dieser Gemüse kann helfen, Entzündungen im Körper zu reduzieren und das Risiko für chronische Krankheiten zu senken.

Ein weiterer zentraler Bestandteil der entzündungshemmenden Ernährung sind Omega-3-Fettsäuren. Diese essenziellen Fette, die hauptsächlich in fettreichem Fisch wie Lachs, Makrele und Hering sowie in Leinsamen, Chiasamen und Walnüssen vorkommen, sind bekannt für ihre Fähigkeit, entzündungsfördernde Substanzen im Körper zu hemmen. Omega-3-Fettsäuren unterstützen die Produktion von entzündungshemmenden Eicosanoiden, die helfen, Entzündungen zu kontrollieren und zu lindern.

Nüsse und Samen spielen ebenfalls eine wichtige Rolle. Mandeln, Walnüsse, Sonnenblumenkerne und Chiasamen liefern nicht nur gesunde Fette, sondern auch eine Vielzahl von Vitaminen und Mineralstoffen, die das Immunsystem stärken und Entzündungen bekämpfen. Der regelmäßige Verzehr von Nüssen und Samen ist mit einem geringeren Risiko für Herzkrankheiten und chronische Entzündungen verbunden.

Die Verwendung von Olivenöl, insbesondere extra nativem Olivenöl, ist ein weiterer Schlüssel zur Reduzierung von Entzündungen. Olivenöl ist reich an einfach ungesättigten Fettsäuren und Antioxidantien, insbesondere Oleocanthal, das ähnliche entzündungshemmende Wirkungen wie Ibuprofen aufweist. Studien haben gezeigt, dass der Konsum von Olivenöl positive Auswirkungen auf die Herzgesundheit hat und Entzündungen im Körper verringert.

Hülsenfrüchte wie Linsen, Kichererbsen und schwarze Bohnen sind hervorragende Quellen für pflanzliches Protein und Ballaststoffe. Sie unterstützen eine gesunde Darmflora, die eine wesentliche Rolle bei der Regulation von Entzündungen spielt. Ballaststoffe fördern das Wachstum nützlicher Darmbakterien, die entzündungshemmende kurzkettige Fettsäuren produzieren.

Gewürze und Kräuter dürfen in einer entzündungshemmenden Ernährung nicht fehlen. Kurkuma, das den Wirkstoff Curcumin enthält, ist ein besonders starkes Entzündungshemmungsmittel. Curcumin hemmt verschiedene Moleküle, die Entzündungen fördern, und wird für seine vielseitigen gesundheitlichen Vorteile geschätzt. Ingwer, der Gingerole enthält, ist ein weiteres Gewürz, das entzündungshemmend wirkt. Die regelmäßige Verwendung von Knoblauch, der Allicin enthält, kann ebenfalls dazu beitragen, Entzündungen zu reduzieren und das Immunsystem zu stärken.

Neben diesen spezifischen Lebensmitteln spielt die Auswahl der Kohlenhydrate eine bedeutende Rolle. Vollkornprodukte wie Hafer, Quinoa, brauner Reis und Dinkel enthalten Ballaststoffe und Nährstoffe, die den Blutzuckerspiegel stabilisieren und Entzündungen verringern können. Raffinierte Kohlenhydrate, wie sie in Weißbrot und zuckerhaltigen Produkten vorkommen, sollten hingegen gemieden werden, da sie Entzündungen fördern können.

Profil der Nährstoffe und ihre Wirkungen

Im Rahmen einer entzündungshemmenden Ernährung spielen bestimmte Nährstoffe eine entscheidende Rolle, da sie die Fähigkeit besitzen, entzündliche Prozesse im Körper zu modulieren und das allgemeine Wohlbefinden zu fördern. Es ist wichtig zu verstehen, wie diese Nährstoffe wirken und warum sie so effektiv sind.

Beginnen wir mit den Omega-3-Fettsäuren, die eine zentrale Rolle in der Bekämpfung von Entzündungen einnehmen. Diese mehrfach ungesättigten Fettsäuren sind in Lebensmitteln wie fettem Fisch (z.B. Lachs, Makrele, Sardinen), Leinsamen, Chiasamen und Walnüssen enthalten. Omega-3-Fettsäuren sind bekannt dafür, die Produktion entzündungsfördernder Substanzen wie Eicosanoide und Zytokine zu hemmen. Sie fördern die Bildung von entzündungshemmenden Molekülen wie Resolvine und Protectine, die helfen, entzündliche Reaktionen zu beenden und die Heilung zu unterstützen.

Antioxidantien sind eine weitere bedeutende Gruppe von Nährstoffen mit starken entzündungshemmenden Eigenschaften. Diese Verbindungen schützen die Zellen vor oxidativem Stress, der durch freie Radikale verursacht wird und zu chronischen Entzündungen führen kann. Vitamin C, das in Zitrusfrüchten, Beeren und grünem Blattgemüse vorkommt, ist ein kraftvolles Antioxidans, das das Immunsystem stärkt und die Heilung von Gewebe fördert. Vitamin E, das in Nüssen, Samen und pflanzlichen Ölen wie Olivenöl enthalten ist, schützt die Zellmembranen vor Schäden und unterstützt die Immunfunktion.

Polyphenole, eine Gruppe sekundärer Pflanzenstoffe, sind ebenfalls für ihre entzündungshemmenden Eigenschaften bekannt. Diese Verbindungen kommen in einer Vielzahl von Lebensmitteln vor, darunter Beeren, Tee, Kaffee, dunkle Schokolade und Trauben. Polyphenole wirken, indem sie entzündungsfördernde Enzyme hemmen und die Expression von Genen beeinflussen, die an entzündlichen Prozessen beteiligt sind. Resveratrol, ein bekanntes Polyphenol in Trauben und Rotwein, hat gezeigt, dass es die Aktivität von NF-kB, einem Schlüsselmolekül in der Entzündungsreaktion, hemmen kann.

Ein weiterer wichtiger Nährstoff in der entzündungshemmenden Ernährung ist das Curcumin, das in Kurkuma enthalten ist. Curcumin hat starke entzündungshemmende und antioxidative Eigenschaften. Es wirkt, indem es die Produktion von proinflammatorischen Molekülen wie Zytokinen und Cyclooxygenase-2 (COX-2) hemmt. Studien haben gezeigt, dass Curcumin bei der Behandlung von entzündlichen Erkrankungen wie Arthritis und Darmentzündungen wirksam sein kann.

Ballaststoffe sind essenziell für eine gesunde Ernährung und spielen eine wichtige Rolle bei der Regulierung von Entzündungen. Sie sind in Vollkornprodukten, Obst, Gemüse, Hülsenfrüchten und Nüssen enthalten. Ballaststoffe fördern eine gesunde Darmflora, die wiederum entzündungshemmende kurzkettige Fettsäuren wie Butyrat produziert. Diese Fettsäuren stärken die Darmbarriere und verhindern das Eindringen von entzündungsfördernden Substanzen in den Körper.

Vitamin D ist ein weiterer Nährstoff, der für seine entzündungshemmenden Wirkungen bekannt ist. Es unterstützt die Regulierung des Immunsystems und hilft, die Produktion von proinflammatorischen Zytokinen zu reduzieren. Ein Mangel an Vitamin D wird mit einem erhöhten Risiko für chronische Entzündungen und Autoimmunerkrankungen in Verbindung gebracht. Quellen für Vitamin D sind fetter Fisch, angereicherte Lebensmittel und Sonneneinstrahlung.

Probiotika, lebende Mikroorganismen, die gesundheitliche Vorteile bieten, sind ebenfalls wichtig für die Entzündungsregulation. Sie fördern eine gesunde Darmflora und modulieren das Immunsystem. Probiotika sind in fermentierten Lebensmitteln wie Joghurt, Sauerkraut, Kimchi und Kefir enthalten. Diese Mikroorganismen unterstützen die Produktion von entzündungshemmenden Substanzen und stärken die Darmbarriere.

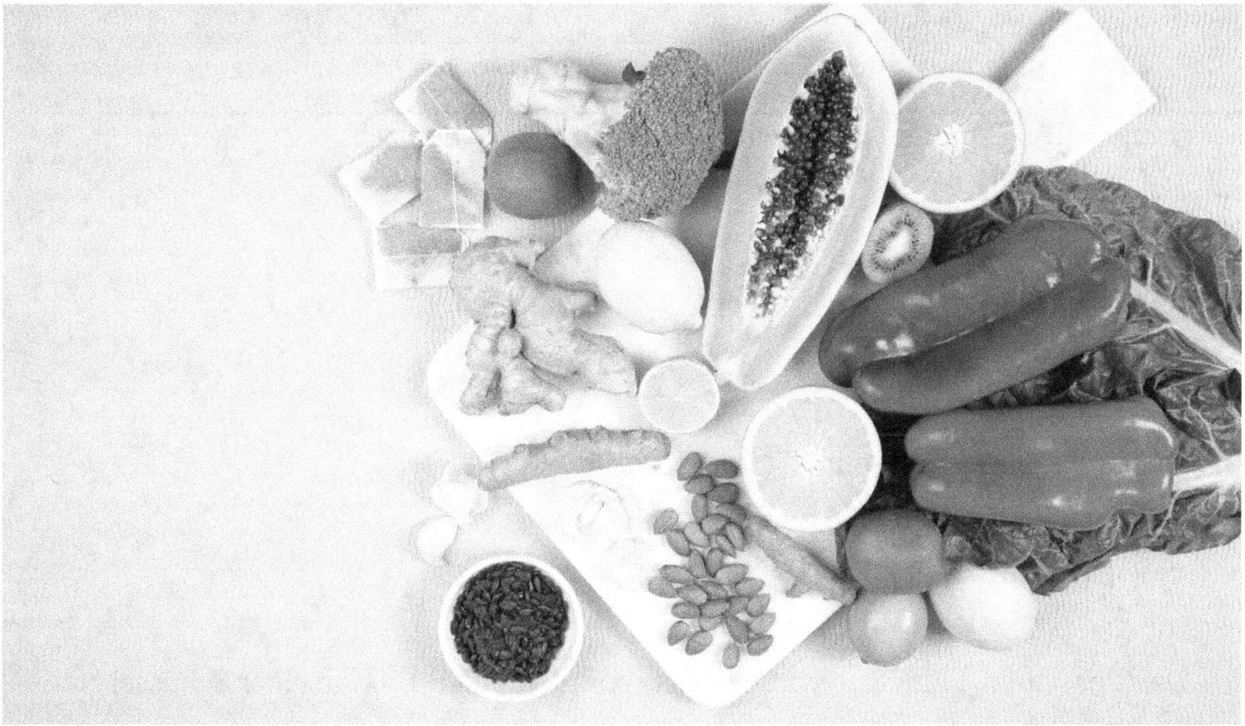

Kapitel 3: Rezepte für das Frühstück

Der Start in den Tag

1. Heidelbeer-Chia-Pudding

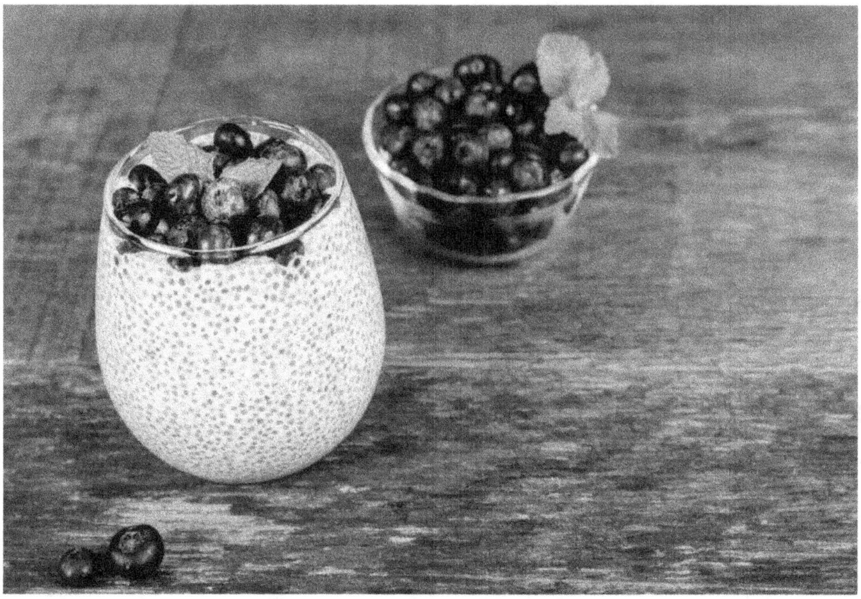

Zubereitungszeit: 10 Minuten | Kochzeit: 0 Minuten | Portionen: 2

Schwierigkeiten: Einfach

Zutaten:

- 4 EL Chiasamen
- 250 ml Mandelmilch
- 1 TL Ahornsirup
- 100 g frische Heidelbeeren
- 1 TL Vanilleextrakt
- 1 EL gehackte Mandeln

Zubereitung:

1. Die Chiasamen, Mandelmilch, Ahornsirup und Vanilleextrakt in einer Schüssel gut verrühren.

2. Die Mischung abdecken und mindestens 4 Stunden oder über Nacht im Kühlschrank quellen lassen.
3. Vor dem Servieren die Heidelbeeren unterheben.
4. In zwei Schalen verteilen und mit gehackten Mandeln garnieren.
5. Sofort servieren und genießen.

Nährwerte (pro Portion): Kalorien: 210 | Fett: 10g | Kohlenhydrate: 20g | Protein: 6g | Zucker: 9g | Natrium: 80mg

2. Avocado-Toast mit Tomaten und Kresse

Zubereitungszeit: 10 Minuten | Kochzeit: 5 Minuten | Portionen: 2

Schwierigkeiten: Einfach

Zutaten:

- 2 Scheiben Vollkornbrot
- 1 reife Avocado
- 1 kleine Tomate, in Scheiben geschnitten
- Eine Handvoll frische Kresse
- 1 EL Zitronensaft
- Salz und Pfeffer nach Geschmack

Zubereitung:

1. Die Avocado halbieren, entkernen und das Fruchtfleisch in einer Schüssel zerdrücken.
2. Zitronensaft, Salz und Pfeffer zur Avocado hinzufügen und gut vermischen.
3. Das Vollkornbrot im Toaster oder in einer Pfanne leicht anrösten.
4. Die Avocadomischung auf die gerösteten Brotscheiben streichen.
5. Mit Tomatenscheiben und frischer Kresse belegen und sofort servieren.

Nährwerte (pro Portion): Kalorien: 250 | Fett: 15g | Kohlenhydrate: 30g | Protein: 5g | Zucker: 2g | Natrium: 150mg

3. Grüner Smoothie mit Spinat und Ananas

Zubereitungszeit: 5 Minuten | Kochzeit: 0 Minuten | Portionen: 2

Schwierigkeiten: Einfach

Zutaten:

- 2 Handvoll frischer Spinat
- 1 Banane
- 200 g frische Ananas
- 300 ml Kokoswasser
- 1 EL Leinsamen

Zubereitung:

1. Den Spinat waschen und gut abtropfen lassen.
2. Die Banane schälen und in Stücke schneiden.
3. Ananas schälen und in kleine Stücke schneiden.
4. Alle Zutaten in einen Mixer geben und zu einem glatten Smoothie pürieren.
5. In zwei Gläser füllen und sofort genießen.

Nährwerte (pro Portion): Kalorien: 180 | Fett: 4g | Kohlenhydrate: 35g | Protein: 3g | Zucker: 20g | Natrium: 60mg

4. Haferflocken mit Apfel und Zimt

Zubereitungszeit: 5 Minuten | Kochzeit: 10 Minuten | Portionen: 2

Schwierigkeiten: Einfach

Zutaten:

- 100 g Haferflocken
- 300 ml Mandelmilch
- 1 Apfel, gewürfelt
- 1 TL Zimt
- 1 EL Walnüsse, gehackt
- 1 TL Ahornsirup

Zubereitung:

1. Die Haferflocken und Mandelmilch in einem Topf bei mittlerer Hitze erwärmen.
2. Den gewürfelten Apfel und den Zimt hinzufügen und gut umrühren.

3. Die Mischung unter ständigem Rühren köcheln lassen, bis die Haferflocken weich sind und die gewünschte Konsistenz erreicht ist.
4. In Schalen füllen, mit gehackten Walnüssen bestreuen und mit Ahornsirup beträufeln.
5. Sofort servieren und genießen.

Nährwerte (pro Portion): Kalorien: 290 | Fett: 9g | Kohlenhydrate: 45g | Protein: 6g | Zucker: 12g | Natrium: 80mg

5. Quinoa-Frühstücksschale mit Beeren

Zubereitungszeit: 10 Minuten | Kochzeit: 15 Minuten | Portionen: 2

Schwierigkeiten: Mittel

Zutaten:

- 100 g Quinoa
- 200 ml Wasser
- 100 g gemischte Beeren (Himbeeren, Heidelbeeren, Erdbeeren)
- 2 EL Mandelblättchen
- 1 TL Ahornsirup
- 1 TL Zimt
- 100 ml Mandelmilch

Zubereitung:

1. Die Quinoa in einem Sieb unter fließendem Wasser abspülen.
2. Wasser und Quinoa in einen Topf geben, zum Kochen bringen, dann die Hitze reduzieren und 15 Minuten köcheln lassen, bis die Quinoa weich ist und das Wasser absorbiert wurde.
3. Die gekochte Quinoa in Schalen füllen und mit Mandelmilch übergießen.
4. Beeren, Mandelblättchen, Ahornsirup und Zimt darauf verteilen.
5. Sofort servieren und genießen.

Nährwerte (pro Portion): Kalorien: 300 | Fett: 10g | Kohlenhydrate: 45g | Protein: 8g | Zucker: 15g | Natrium: 40mg

6. Mandel- und Blaubeer-Muffins

Zubereitungszeit: 15 Minuten | Kochzeit: 25 Minuten | Portionen: 2

Schwierigkeiten: Mittel

Zutaten:

- 150 g Mandelmehl
- 50 g Haferflocken
- 1 TL Backpulver
- 2 Eier
- 2 EL Kokosöl, geschmolzen
- 2 EL Ahornsirup
- 100 g frische Blaubeeren
- 1 TL Vanilleextrakt

Zubereitung:

1. Den Ofen auf 180 Grad vorheizen und ein Muffinblech mit Papierförmchen auslegen.
2. Mandelmehl, Haferflocken und Backpulver in einer Schüssel vermischen.
3. Eier, geschmolzenes Kokosöl, Ahornsirup und Vanilleextrakt in einer separaten Schüssel verrühren.
4. Die feuchten Zutaten zu den trockenen Zutaten geben und gut vermischen.
5. Blaubeeren unterheben und den Teig in die Muffinformen füllen.
6. 25 Minuten backen, bis die Muffins goldbraun sind und ein Zahnstocher sauber herauskommt.

Nährwerte (pro Portion): Kalorien: 250 | Fett: 15g | Kohlenhydrate: 20g | Protein: 7g | Zucker: 10g | Natrium: 90mg

7. Buchweizen-Pfannkuchen mit Beerenkompott

Zubereitungszeit: 10 Minuten | Kochzeit: 20 Minuten | Portionen: 2

Schwierigkeiten: Mittel

Zutaten:

- 100 g Buchweizenmehl
- 1 TL Backpulver
- 1 Ei
- 200 ml Mandelmilch

- 1 TL Vanilleextrakt
- 100 g gemischte Beeren
- 1 EL Ahornsirup

Zubereitung:

1. Buchweizenmehl und Backpulver in einer Schüssel vermischen.
2. Ei, Mandelmilch und Vanilleextrakt hinzufügen und zu einem glatten Teig verrühren.
3. Eine Pfanne erhitzen und den Teig portionsweise hineingeben, Pfannkuchen von beiden Seiten goldbraun backen.
4. In einem kleinen Topf die Beeren mit dem Ahornsirup erhitzen, bis ein Kompott entsteht.
5. Die Pfannkuchen mit dem Beerenkompott servieren und genießen.

Nährwerte (pro Portion): Kalorien: 220 | Fett: 6g | Kohlenhydrate: 35g | Protein: 6g | Zucker: 10g | Natrium: 70mg

8. Kokosnuss-Granola mit Joghurt

Zubereitungszeit: 10 Minuten | Kochzeit: 20 Minuten | Portionen: 2

Schwierigkeiten: Einfach

Zutaten:

- 100 g Haferflocken
- 50 g Kokosraspeln
- 30 g gehackte Mandeln
- 2 EL Kokosöl, geschmolzen
- 2 EL Ahornsirup
- 200 g griechischer Joghurt
- 1 TL Zimt

Zubereitung:

1. Den Ofen auf 180 Grad vorheizen und ein Backblech mit Backpapier auslegen.
2. Haferflocken, Kokosraspeln und Mandeln in einer Schüssel vermischen.
3. Geschmolzenes Kokosöl und Ahornsirup hinzufügen und gut verrühren.
4. Die Mischung gleichmäßig auf dem Backblech verteilen und 20 Minuten backen, dabei gelegentlich umrühren.
5. Das fertige Granola mit griechischem Joghurt und Zimt servieren.

Nährwerte (pro Portion): Kalorien: 350 | Fett: 18g | Kohlenhydrate: 35g | Protein: 10g | Zucker: 12g | Natrium: 80mg

9. Bircher Müsli

Zubereitungszeit: 10 Minuten | Kochzeit: 0 Minuten | Portionen: 2

Schwierigkeiten: Einfach

Zutaten:

- 100 g Haferflocken
- 200 ml Mandelmilch
- 1 Apfel, gerieben
- 2 EL Rosinen
- 1 EL Chiasamen
- 1 TL Zimt
- 50 g gehackte Nüsse

Zubereitung:

1. Haferflocken, Mandelmilch, geriebener Apfel, Rosinen, Chiasamen und Zimt in einer Schüssel vermischen.
2. Abdecken und über Nacht im Kühlschrank quellen lassen.
3. Vor dem Servieren die gehackten Nüsse unterheben.
4. In Schalen verteilen und sofort genießen.

Nährwerte (pro Portion): Kalorien: 280 | Fett: 10g | Kohlenhydrate: 45g | Protein: 6g | Zucker: 15g | Natrium: 60mg

10. Süßkartoffel-Toast mit Avocado und Ei

Zubereitungszeit: 10 Minuten | Kochzeit: 15 Minuten | Portionen: 2

Schwierigkeiten: Mittel

Zutaten:

- 1 große Süßkartoffel
- 1 reife Avocado
- 2 Eier
- 1 EL Zitronensaft
- Salz und Pfeffer nach Geschmack
- Eine Handvoll Kresse

Zubereitung:

1. Die Süßkartoffel in etwa 1 cm dicke Scheiben schneiden und im Toaster rösten, bis sie weich sind.
2. Die Avocado halbieren, entkernen und das Fruchtfleisch in einer Schüssel zerdrücken.
3. Zitronensaft, Salz und Pfeffer zur Avocado hinzufügen und gut vermischen.
4. Die Eier in einem Topf mit kochendem Wasser etwa 5-7 Minuten kochen, bis sie weichgekocht sind.
5. Die Süßkartoffel-Scheiben mit der Avocadomischung bestreichen, die Eier darauflegen, mit Kresse garnieren und sofort servieren.

Nährwerte (pro Portion): Kalorien: 300 | Fett: 15g | Kohlenhydrate: 35g | Protein: 8g | Zucker: 5g | Natrium: 90mg

Nährstoffreiche Frühstücksvarianten

11. Matcha-Grüner-Smoothie-Bowl

Zubereitungszeit: 10 Minuten | Kochzeit: 0 Minuten | Portionen: 2

Schwierigkeiten: Einfach

Zutaten:

- 2 reife Bananen, gefroren
- 1 Handvoll Spinat
- 1 TL Matcha-Pulver
- 200 ml Mandelmilch
- 1 TL Chiasamen
- 1 TL Ahornsirup
- 1 Kiwi, geschält und in Scheiben geschnitten
- 1 EL Granola

Zubereitung:

1. Die gefrorenen Bananen, Spinat, Matcha-Pulver, Mandelmilch und Ahornsirup in einen Mixer geben und zu einer glatten Masse pürieren.
2. Die Mischung in Schalen füllen.
3. Mit Kiwi-Scheiben, Chiasamen und Granola garnieren.
4. Sofort servieren und genießen.

Nährwerte (pro Portion): Kalorien: 250 | Fett: 6g | Kohlenhydrate: 45g | Protein: 5g | Zucker: 20g | Natrium: 50mg

12. Quinoa-Obstsalat

Zubereitungszeit: 15 Minuten | Kochzeit: 15 Minuten | Portionen: 2

Schwierigkeiten: Einfach

Zutaten:

- 100 g Quinoa
- 200 ml Wasser
- 1 Apfel, gewürfelt
- 1 Orange, geschält und in Stücke geschnitten

- 1 Kiwi, geschält und in Scheiben geschnitten
- 1 Handvoll Trauben, halbiert
- 1 TL Zimt
- 1 EL Ahornsirup
- 2 EL gehackte Mandeln

Zubereitung:

1. Die Quinoa in einem Sieb abspülen.
2. Wasser und Quinoa in einem Topf zum Kochen bringen, dann die Hitze reduzieren und 15 Minuten köcheln lassen, bis die Quinoa weich ist und das Wasser absorbiert wurde.
3. Die Quinoa abkühlen lassen.
4. Das Obst in eine große Schüssel geben, die abgekühlte Quinoa, Zimt und Ahornsirup hinzufügen und gut vermischen.
5. Mit gehackten Mandeln bestreuen und servieren.

Nährwerte (pro Portion): Kalorien: 300 | Fett: 8g | Kohlenhydrate: 55g | Protein: 7g | Zucker: 20g | Natrium: 20mg

13. Süßkartoffel- und Avocado-Brei

Zubereitungszeit: 10 Minuten | Kochzeit: 10 Minuten | Portionen: 2

Schwierigkeiten: Mittel

Zutaten:

- 1 große Süßkartoffel, geschält und gewürfelt
- 1 reife Avocado
- 200 ml Mandelmilch
- 1 TL Zimt
- 1 EL Kokosflocken
- 1 TL Honig

Zubereitung:

1. Die Süßkartoffelwürfel in einem Topf mit Wasser zum Kochen bringen und weich kochen.
2. Die gekochten Süßkartoffeln abtropfen lassen und in eine Schüssel geben.
3. Die Avocado halbieren, entkernen und das Fruchtfleisch zu den Süßkartoffeln geben.
4. Mandelmilch und Zimt hinzufügen und alles zu einer cremigen Masse pürieren.
5. Mit Kokosflocken und Honig garnieren und servieren.

Nährwerte (pro Portion): Kalorien: 320 | Fett: 15g | Kohlenhydrate: 40g | Protein: 4g | Zucker: 10g | Natrium: 40mg

14. Hirsebrei mit Beeren

Zubereitungszeit: 10 Minuten | Kochzeit: 15 Minuten | Portionen: 2

Schwierigkeiten: Einfach

Zutaten:

- 100 g Hirse
- 300 ml Mandelmilch
- 1 TL Zimt
- 1 TL Vanilleextrakt
- 100 g gemischte Beeren (Erdbeeren, Himbeeren, Heidelbeeren)
- 1 EL gehackte Mandeln
- 1 EL Ahornsirup

Zubereitung:

1. Die Hirse in einem Sieb abspülen.
2. Mandelmilch in einem Topf zum Kochen bringen, Hirse hinzufügen und 15 Minuten köcheln lassen, bis die Hirse weich ist und die Milch absorbiert wurde.
3. Zimt und Vanilleextrakt unterrühren.
4. Den Hirsebrei in Schalen füllen und mit Beeren, gehackten Mandeln und Ahornsirup garnieren.
5. Sofort servieren und genießen.

Nährwerte (pro Portion): Kalorien: 270 | Fett: 8g | Kohlenhydrate: 45g | Protein: 6g | Zucker: 15g | Natrium: 30mg

15. Mandel- und Kokos-Joghurtparfait

Zubereitungszeit: 10 Minuten | Kochzeit: 0 Minuten | Portionen: 2

Schwierigkeiten: Einfach

Zutaten:

- 200 g Kokosjoghurt
- 50 g Mandeln, gehackt
- 50 g frische Himbeeren

- 50 g frische Heidelbeeren
- 1 EL Chiasamen
- 1 EL Honig

Zubereitung:

1. Den Kokosjoghurt gleichmäßig auf zwei Gläser verteilen.
2. Gehackte Mandeln, Himbeeren, Heidelbeeren und Chiasamen schichtenweise darüber geben.
3. Mit einem Teelöffel Honig beträufeln.
4. Das Parfait sofort servieren oder im Kühlschrank aufbewahren.
5. Optional kann man es mit ein paar Minzblättern garnieren.

Nährwerte (pro Portion): Kalorien: 280 | Fett: 15g | Kohlenhydrate: 25g | Protein: 6g | Zucker: 12g | Natrium: 30mg

16. Zucchini- und Möhrenpuffer

Zubereitungszeit: 15 Minuten | Kochzeit: 10 Minuten | Portionen: 2

Schwierigkeiten: Mittel

Zutaten:

- 1 Zucchini, geraspelt
- 1 Karotte, geraspelt
- 2 Eier
- 2 EL Vollkornmehl
- 1 TL Kreuzkümmel
- Salz und Pfeffer nach Geschmack
- 2 EL Olivenöl
- 2 EL griechischer Joghurt
- 1 TL Zitronensaft

Zubereitung:

1. Zucchini und Karotte in eine Schüssel geben und überschüssige Flüssigkeit ausdrücken.
2. Eier, Mehl, Kreuzkümmel, Salz und Pfeffer hinzufügen und gut vermischen.
3. Olivenöl in einer Pfanne erhitzen und die Mischung löffelweise in die Pfanne geben, flachdrücken und von beiden Seiten goldbraun braten.
4. Die Puffer auf Küchenpapier abtropfen lassen.
5. Mit einem Klecks Joghurt und Zitronensaft servieren.

Nährwerte (pro Portion): Kalorien: 200 | Fett: 10g | Kohlenhydrate: 20g | Protein: 7g | Zucker: 4g | Natrium: 70mg

17. Chia-Pudding mit Mango und Kokos

Zubereitungszeit: 10 Minuten | Kochzeit: 0 Minuten | Portionen: 2

Schwierigkeiten: Einfach

Zutaten:

- 4 EL Chiasamen
- 250 ml Kokosmilch
- 1 TL Vanilleextrakt
- 1 reife Mango, gewürfelt
- 1 EL Kokosflocken

Zubereitung:

1. Chiasamen, Kokosmilch und Vanilleextrakt in einer Schüssel gut verrühren.
2. Abdecken und über Nacht im Kühlschrank quellen lassen.
3. Vor dem Servieren die Mango über den Chia-Pudding verteilen.
4. Mit Kokosflocken bestreuen und genießen.

Nährwerte (pro Portion): Kalorien: 260 | Fett: 15g | Kohlenhydrate: 30g | Protein: 5g | Zucker: 15g | Natrium: 20mg

18. Buchweizen-Müsli mit Äpfeln und Nüssen

Zubereitungszeit: 10 Minuten | Kochzeit: 5 Minuten | Portionen: 2

Schwierigkeiten: Einfach

Zutaten:

- 100 g Buchweizenflocken
- 1 Apfel, geraspelt
- 2 EL Rosinen
- 2 EL gehackte Haselnüsse
- 200 ml Mandelmilch
- 1 TL Zimt
- 1 TL Honig

Zubereitung:

1. Buchweizenflocken in eine Schüssel geben.
2. Geraspelten Apfel, Rosinen und gehackte Haselnüsse hinzufügen.
3. Mandelmilch und Zimt unterrühren.
4. Mit einem Teelöffel Honig abschmecken.
5. Sofort servieren und genießen.

Nährwerte (pro Portion): Kalorien: 250 | Fett: 8g | Kohlenhydrate: 40g | Protein: 5g | Zucker: 15g | Natrium: 25mg

19. Hummus-Toast mit Paprika und Kresse

Zubereitungszeit: 10 Minuten | Kochzeit: 5 Minuten | Portionen: 2

Schwierigkeiten: Einfach

Zutaten:

- 2 Scheiben Vollkornbrot
- 4 EL Hummus
- 1 rote Paprika, in Streifen geschnitten
- Eine Handvoll frische Kresse
- 1 EL Olivenöl
- Salz und Pfeffer nach Geschmack

Zubereitung:

1. Das Vollkornbrot im Toaster leicht anrösten.
2. Hummus gleichmäßig auf die Brotscheiben streichen.
3. Paprikastreifen und Kresse darauf verteilen.
4. Mit einem Spritzer Olivenöl beträufeln und mit Salz und Pfeffer würzen.
5. Sofort servieren und genießen.

Nährwerte (pro Portion): Kalorien: 280 | Fett: 12g | Kohlenhydrate: 35g | Protein: 7g | Zucker: 4g | Natrium: 140mg

20. Tofu-Rührei mit Spinat und Tomaten

Zubereitungszeit: 10 Minuten | Kochzeit: 10 Minuten | Portionen: 2

Schwierigkeiten: Mittel

Zutaten:

- 200 g Tofu, zerkrümelt
- 1 Handvoll frischer Spinat
- 1 Tomate, gewürfelt
- 1 kleine Zwiebel, fein gehackt
- 1 EL Olivenöl
- 1 TL Kurkuma
- Salz und Pfeffer nach Geschmack

Zubereitung:

1. Olivenöl in einer Pfanne erhitzen und die gehackte Zwiebel darin anbraten, bis sie weich ist.
2. Zerkrümelten Tofu, Kurkuma, Salz und Pfeffer hinzufügen und gut vermischen.
3. Den Tofu anbraten, bis er leicht gebräunt ist.
4. Spinat und gewürfelte Tomate hinzufügen und weiterkochen, bis der Spinat zusammengefallen ist.
5. Sofort servieren und genießen.

Nährwerte (pro Portion): Kalorien: 220 | Fett: 12g | Kohlenhydrate: 15g | Protein: 15g | Zucker: 5g | Natrium: 150mg

Kapitel 4: Rezepte für das Mittagessen

Energie für das Mittagessen

21. Quinoa-Gemüse-Bowl

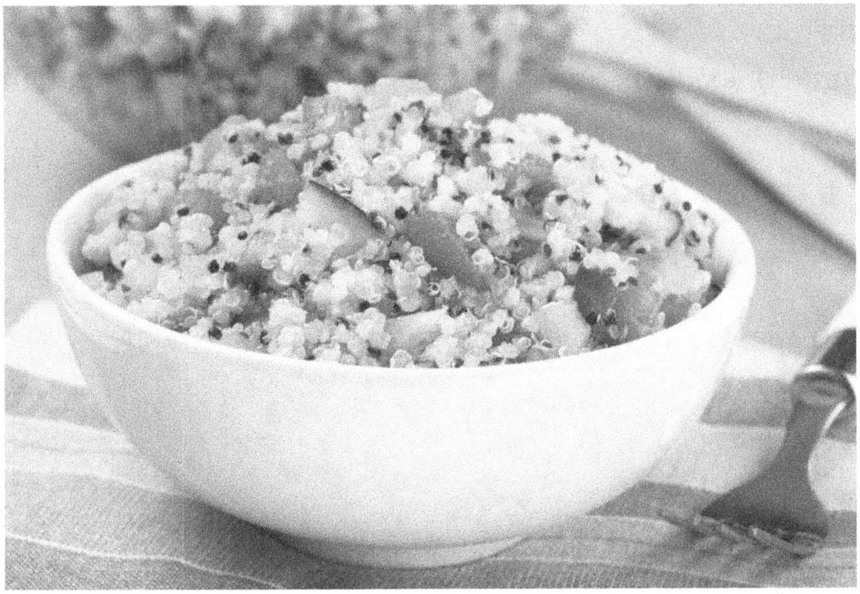

Zubereitungszeit: 15 Minuten | Kochzeit: 15 Minuten | Portionen: 2

Schwierigkeiten: Mittel

Zutaten:

- 100 g Quinoa
- 200 ml Gemüsebrühe
- 1 kleine Zucchini, gewürfelt
- 1 rote Paprika, gewürfelt
- 1 Karotte, in Streifen geschnitten
- 1 Handvoll Spinat
- 1 Avocado, in Scheiben
- 1 EL Zitronensaft
- Salz und Pfeffer nach Geschmack

Zubereitung:

1. Die Quinoa in einem Sieb abspülen und mit der Gemüsebrühe in einem Topf zum Kochen bringen. 15 Minuten köcheln lassen, bis die Quinoa weich ist und die Flüssigkeit absorbiert wurde.
2. In einer Pfanne die Zucchini, Paprika und Karotten bei mittlerer Hitze unter gelegentlichem Rühren anbraten.
3. Den Spinat hinzufügen und unter Rühren kochen, bis er zusammenfällt.
4. Die gekochte Quinoa in zwei Schalen verteilen und das gebratene Gemüse darüber geben.
5. Mit Avocadoscheiben garnieren, mit Zitronensaft beträufeln und mit Salz und Pfeffer abschmecken.

Nährwerte (pro Portion): Kalorien: 320 | Fett: 15g | Kohlenhydrate: 40g | Protein: 8g | Zucker: 7g | Natrium: 200mg

22. Linsensalat mit Rote Bete und Walnüssen

Zubereitungszeit: 10 Minuten | Kochzeit: 20 Minuten | Portionen: 2

Schwierigkeiten: Mittel

Zutaten:

- 150 g grüne Linsen
- 2 mittelgroße Rote Bete, gekocht und gewürfelt
- 1 kleine rote Zwiebel, fein gehackt
- 50 g Walnüsse, grob gehackt
- 1 Handvoll Rucola
- 2 EL Apfelessig
- 1 EL Olivenöl (nicht erhitzt)
- Salz und Pfeffer nach Geschmack

Zubereitung:

1. Die Linsen in einem Topf mit Wasser zum Kochen bringen und 20 Minuten köcheln lassen, bis sie weich sind. Abgießen und abkühlen lassen.
2. In einer großen Schüssel die gekochten Linsen, gewürfelte Rote Bete, gehackte Zwiebel und Walnüsse vermischen.
3. Rucola hinzufügen und vorsichtig unterheben.
4. Apfelessig und Olivenöl über den Salat geben, gut vermischen und mit Salz und Pfeffer abschmecken.
5. Sofort servieren oder im Kühlschrank aufbewahren.

Nährwerte (pro Portion): Kalorien: 280 | Fett: 14g | Kohlenhydrate: 30g | Protein: 10g | Zucker: 6g | Natrium: 150mg

23. Kichererbsen-Curry mit Spinat

Zubereitungszeit: 15 Minuten | Kochzeit: 25 Minuten | Portionen: 2

Schwierigkeiten: Mittel

Zutaten:

- 1 Dose Kichererbsen (400 g), abgetropft und gespült
- 200 g frischer Spinat
- 1 Zwiebel, gehackt
- 2 Knoblauchzehen, gehackt
- 1 Stück Ingwer (ca. 2 cm), gerieben
- 1 Dose Kokosmilch (400 ml)
- 2 EL Tomatenmark
- 1 TL Kurkuma
- 1 TL Kreuzkümmel
- 1 TL Koriander
- Salz und Pfeffer nach Geschmack

Zubereitung:

1. In einem großen Topf die gehackte Zwiebel, Knoblauch und geriebenen Ingwer bei mittlerer Hitze unter Rühren anbraten, bis die Zwiebel weich ist.
2. Kurkuma, Kreuzkümmel und Koriander hinzufügen und kurz mit anrösten.
3. Tomatenmark unterrühren und die Kichererbsen dazugeben.
4. Kokosmilch einrühren und das Curry bei niedriger Hitze etwa 20 Minuten köcheln lassen.
5. Den Spinat hinzufügen und unter Rühren kochen, bis er zusammenfällt. Mit Salz und Pfeffer abschmecken.

Nährwerte (pro Portion): Kalorien: 350 | Fett: 18g | Kohlenhydrate: 35g | Protein: 12g | Zucker: 8g | Natrium: 200mg

24. Gebackene Süßkartoffel mit Avocado-Salsa

Zubereitungszeit: 10 Minuten | Kochzeit: 40 Minuten | Portionen: 2

Schwierigkeiten: Mittel

Zutaten:

- 2 große Süßkartoffeln
- 1 reife Avocado, gewürfelt
- 1 Tomate, gewürfelt
- 1 kleine rote Zwiebel, fein gehackt
- 1 EL frischer Koriander, gehackt
- 1 EL Limettensaft
- Salz und Pfeffer nach Geschmack

Zubereitung:

1. Den Ofen auf 200 Grad vorheizen.
2. Die Süßkartoffeln waschen, trocknen und mit einer Gabel ein paar Mal einstechen. Auf ein Backblech legen und 40 Minuten backen, bis sie weich sind.
3. Während die Süßkartoffeln backen, die Avocado, Tomate, Zwiebel und Koriander in einer Schüssel vermischen.
4. Limettensaft hinzufügen und mit Salz und Pfeffer abschmecken.
5. Die gebackenen Süßkartoffeln längs aufschneiden und die Avocado-Salsa darüber geben.

Nährwerte (pro Portion): Kalorien: 320 | Fett: 14g | Kohlenhydrate: 45g | Protein: 4g | Zucker: 9g | Natrium: 60mg

25. Mediterrane Kichererbsen-Bowl

Zubereitungszeit: 15 Minuten | Kochzeit: 15 Minuten | Portionen: 2

Schwierigkeiten: Mittel

Zutaten:

- 1 Dose Kichererbsen (400 g), abgetropft und gespült
- 1 Gurke, gewürfelt
- 1 rote Paprika, gewürfelt
- 100 g Kirschtomaten, halbiert
- 1 kleine rote Zwiebel, fein gehackt
- 1 Handvoll Petersilie, gehackt

- 50 g Feta-Käse, zerbröselt
- 2 EL Zitronensaft
- 1 EL Olivenöl (nicht erhitzt)
- Salz und Pfeffer nach Geschmack

Zubereitung:

1. Die Kichererbsen in einer Schüssel mit Gurke, Paprika, Kirschtomaten, Zwiebel und Petersilie vermischen.
2. Feta-Käse hinzufügen und vorsichtig unterheben.
3. Zitronensaft und Olivenöl darüber träufeln und mit Salz und Pfeffer abschmecken.
4. Alles gut vermischen und sofort servieren.

Nährwerte (pro Portion): Kalorien: 290 | Fett: 12g | Kohlenhydrate: 35g | Protein: 10g | Zucker: 7g | Natrium: 250mg

26. Blumenkohl-Reis mit Erbsen und Minze

Zubereitungszeit: 10 Minuten | Kochzeit: 10 Minuten | Portionen: 2

Schwierigkeiten: Einfach

Zutaten:

- 1 kleiner Blumenkohl, in Röschen zerteilt
- 100 g Erbsen, frisch oder gefroren
- 1 Handvoll frische Minzblätter, gehackt
- 1 Knoblauchzehe, gehackt
- 1 EL Zitronensaft
- Salz und Pfeffer nach Geschmack

Zubereitung:

1. Den Blumenkohl in einer Küchenmaschine zu feinen Krümeln verarbeiten.
2. In einer Pfanne den gehackten Knoblauch bei mittlerer Hitze anbraten, bis er duftet.
3. Den Blumenkohlreis hinzufügen und 5-7 Minuten unter Rühren kochen, bis er weich ist.
4. Die Erbsen hinzufügen und weitere 3 Minuten kochen.
5. Mit Zitronensaft, Salz und Pfeffer abschmecken und mit gehackter Minze bestreuen.

Nährwerte (pro Portion): Kalorien: 180 | Fett: 4g | Kohlenhydrate: 25g | Protein: 8g | Zucker: 6g | Natrium: 50mg

27. Tofu-Gemüse-Pfanne

Zubereitungszeit: 15 Minuten | Kochzeit: 15 Minuten | Portionen: 2

Schwierigkeiten: Mittel

Zutaten:

- 200 g Tofu, in Würfel geschnitten
- 1 Zucchini, gewürfelt
- 1 rote Paprika, gewürfelt
- 1 Karotte, in dünne Streifen geschnitten
- 1 Handvoll Spinat
- 2 EL Sojasauce (natriumarm)
- 1 EL Sesamöl (nicht erhitzt)
- 1 TL Ingwer, gerieben
- 1 TL Knoblauch, gehackt
- 1 TL Sesamsamen

Zubereitung:

1. Tofu-Würfel in einer Pfanne bei mittlerer Hitze anbraten, bis sie goldbraun sind.
2. Ingwer und Knoblauch hinzufügen und kurz mit anbraten.
3. Zucchini, Paprika und Karotte in die Pfanne geben und 5-7 Minuten unter Rühren kochen.
4. Spinat hinzufügen und weiterkochen, bis er zusammenfällt.
5. Mit Sojasauce und Sesamöl abschmecken, mit Sesamsamen bestreuen und servieren.

Nährwerte (pro Portion): Kalorien: 250 | Fett: 12g | Kohlenhydrate: 20g | Protein: 15g | Zucker: 6g | Natrium: 400mg

28. Quinoa-Tabouleh mit Granatapfel

Zubereitungszeit: 15 Minuten | Kochzeit: 15 Minuten | Portionen: 2

Schwierigkeiten: Mittel

Zutaten:

- 100 g Quinoa
- 200 ml Wasser
- 1 Granatapfel, entkernt
- 1 Gurke, gewürfelt

- 1 Tomate, gewürfelt
- 1 Handvoll frische Minze, gehackt
- 1 Handvoll Petersilie, gehackt
- 2 EL Zitronensaft
- 1 EL Olivenöl (nicht erhitzt)
- Salz und Pfeffer nach Geschmack

Zubereitung:

1. Die Quinoa in einem Sieb abspülen und mit Wasser in einem Topf zum Kochen bringen. 15 Minuten köcheln lassen, bis die Quinoa weich ist und das Wasser absorbiert wurde. Abkühlen lassen.
2. Die abgekühlte Quinoa in eine große Schüssel geben und mit Granatapfelkernen, Gurke, Tomate, Minze und Petersilie vermischen.
3. Zitronensaft und Olivenöl hinzufügen und gut vermischen.
4. Mit Salz und Pfeffer abschmecken und servieren.

Nährwerte (pro Portion): Kalorien: 320 | Fett: 12g | Kohlenhydrate: 45g | Protein: 8g | Zucker: 14g | Natrium: 60mg

29. Vegane Linsensuppe

Zubereitungszeit: 10 Minuten | Kochzeit: 30 Minuten | Portionen: 2

Schwierigkeiten: Einfach

Zutaten:

- 150 g rote Linsen
- 1 Zwiebel, gehackt
- 2 Karotten, gewürfelt
- 2 Selleriestangen, gewürfelt
- 2 Knoblauchzehen, gehackt
- 1 Dose Tomaten (400 g)
- 1 Liter Gemüsebrühe
- 1 TL Kreuzkümmel
- 1 TL Koriander
- 1 TL Paprika
- Salz und Pfeffer nach Geschmack
- 1 Handvoll frische Petersilie, gehackt

Zubereitung:

1. Die Zwiebel, Karotten, Sellerie und Knoblauch in einem großen Topf bei mittlerer Hitze anbraten, bis das Gemüse weich ist.
2. Kreuzkümmel, Koriander und Paprika hinzufügen und kurz mit anrösten.
3. Tomaten, Linsen und Gemüsebrühe hinzufügen und zum Kochen bringen.
4. Die Hitze reduzieren und die Suppe 25-30 Minuten köcheln lassen, bis die Linsen weich sind.
5. Mit Salz und Pfeffer abschmecken, Petersilie unterrühren und servieren.

Nährwerte (pro Portion): Kalorien: 290 | Fett: 5g | Kohlenhydrate: 45g | Protein: 18g | Zucker: 12g | Natrium: 400mg

30. Gebackene Aubergine mit Tomaten und Tahini

Zubereitungszeit: 10 Minuten | Kochzeit: 35 Minuten | Portionen: 2

Schwierigkeiten: Mittel

Zutaten:

- 2 mittelgroße Auberginen, längs halbiert
- 2 Tomaten, gewürfelt
- 2 EL Tahini
- 1 EL Zitronensaft
- 1 Knoblauchzehe, gehackt
- 1 EL frische Petersilie, gehackt
- Salz und Pfeffer nach Geschmack

Zubereitung:

1. Den Ofen auf 200 Grad vorheizen.
2. Die Auberginenhälften mit einem Messer einschneiden und auf ein Backblech legen.
3. Die Auberginen 30 Minuten backen, bis sie weich sind.
4. In einer kleinen Schüssel Tahini, Zitronensaft, Knoblauch, Salz und Pfeffer vermischen.
5. Die gebackenen Auberginen mit Tomaten und Tahini-Sauce belegen und mit gehackter Petersilie bestreuen.

Nährwerte (pro Portion): Kalorien: 260 | Fett: 14g | Kohlenhydrate: 30g | Protein: 6g | Zucker: 10g | Natrium: 50mg

Leichte und heilsame Gerichte

31. Sommerlicher Gemüsesalat mit Zitronen-Dressing

Zubereitungszeit: 15 Minuten | Kochzeit: 0 Minuten | Portionen: 2

Schwierigkeiten: Einfach

Zutaten:

- 1 Gurke, gewürfelt
- 2 Tomaten, gewürfelt
- 1 gelbe Paprika, gewürfelt
- 1 rote Zwiebel, fein gehackt
- 1 Handvoll Petersilie, gehackt
- 1 Avocado, gewürfelt
- 2 EL Zitronensaft
- 1 EL Olivenöl (nicht erhitzt)
- Salz und Pfeffer nach Geschmack

Zubereitung:

1. Gurke, Tomaten, Paprika, Zwiebel und Petersilie in eine große Schüssel geben und vermischen.
2. Avocado hinzufügen und vorsichtig unterheben.
3. Zitronensaft und Olivenöl hinzufügen und mit Salz und Pfeffer abschmecken.
4. Alles gut vermischen und sofort servieren.

Nährwerte (pro Portion): Kalorien: 220 | Fett: 14g | Kohlenhydrate: 20g | Protein: 4g | Zucker: 7g | Natrium: 50mg

32. Zucchini-Nudeln mit Pesto

Zubereitungszeit: 15 Minuten | Kochzeit: 5 Minuten | Portionen: 2

Schwierigkeiten: Einfach

Zutaten:

- 2 große Zucchini, spiralförmig geschnitten
- 1 Handvoll frisches Basilikum
- 1 Knoblauchzehe

- 2 EL Pinienkerne
- 3 EL Olivenöl (nicht erhitzt)
- 2 EL Zitronensaft
- Salz und Pfeffer nach Geschmack

Zubereitung:

1. Die Zucchini-Nudeln mit etwas Salz bestreuen und 10 Minuten ziehen lassen, um überschüssige Feuchtigkeit zu entfernen.
2. Basilikum, Knoblauch, Pinienkerne, Olivenöl, Zitronensaft, Salz und Pfeffer in einem Mixer zu einem glatten Pesto pürieren.
3. Die Zucchini-Nudeln abtropfen lassen und in eine große Schüssel geben.
4. Das Pesto über die Zucchini-Nudeln geben und gut vermischen.
5. Sofort servieren.

Nährwerte (pro Portion): Kalorien: 200 | Fett: 16g | Kohlenhydrate: 10g | Protein: 4g | Zucker: 4g | Natrium: 60mg

33. Gebackene Paprika mit Quinoa-Füllung

Zubereitungszeit: 20 Minuten | Kochzeit: 30 Minuten | Portionen: 2

Schwierigkeiten: Mittel

Zutaten:

- 2 rote Paprika, halbiert und entkernt
- 100 g Quinoa
- 200 ml Gemüsebrühe
- 1 kleine Zucchini, gewürfelt
- 1 Karotte, gewürfelt
- 1 kleine rote Zwiebel, gehackt
- 2 Knoblauchzehen, gehackt
- 1 Handvoll Petersilie, gehackt
- 2 EL Zitronensaft
- Salz und Pfeffer nach Geschmack

Zubereitung:

1. Die Quinoa in einem Sieb abspülen und mit der Gemüsebrühe in einem Topf zum Kochen bringen. 15 Minuten köcheln lassen, bis die Quinoa weich ist und die Flüssigkeit absorbiert wurde.

2. Zucchini, Karotte, Zwiebel und Knoblauch in einer Pfanne bei mittlerer Hitze anbraten, bis das Gemüse weich ist.
3. Die gekochte Quinoa und das gebratene Gemüse in einer Schüssel vermischen, Petersilie und Zitronensaft hinzufügen und mit Salz und Pfeffer abschmecken.
4. Die Paprikahälften mit der Quinoa-Gemüse-Mischung füllen und in eine Auflaufform legen.
5. Im vorgeheizten Ofen bei 180 Grad 30 Minuten backen, bis die Paprika weich sind.

Nährwerte (pro Portion): Kalorien: 280 | Fett: 8g | Kohlenhydrate: 40g | Protein: 8g | Zucker: 10g | Natrium: 60mg

34. Blumenkohl-Steak mit Tahini-Dressing

Zubereitungszeit: 10 Minuten | Kochzeit: 30 Minuten | Portionen: 2

Schwierigkeiten: Mittel

Zutaten:

- 1 großer Blumenkohl, in 2 dicke Scheiben geschnitten
- 2 EL Olivenöl (nicht erhitzt)
- 1 TL Paprika
- 1 TL Kreuzkümmel
- Salz und Pfeffer nach Geschmack
- 2 EL Tahini
- 1 EL Zitronensaft
- 1 Knoblauchzehe, gehackt
- 2-3 EL Wasser

Zubereitung:

1. Den Ofen auf 200 Grad vorheizen.
2. Die Blumenkohl-Steaks mit Olivenöl bestreichen und mit Paprika, Kreuzkümmel, Salz und Pfeffer würzen.
3. Die Steaks auf ein Backblech legen und 30 Minuten backen, bis sie goldbraun und zart sind.
4. Währenddessen Tahini, Zitronensaft, Knoblauch und Wasser in einer kleinen Schüssel verrühren, bis ein glattes Dressing entsteht.
5. Die Blumenkohl-Steaks mit dem Tahini-Dressing servieren.

Nährwerte (pro Portion): Kalorien: 200 | Fett: 12g | Kohlenhydrate: 18g | Protein: 6g | Zucker: 5g | Natrium: 150mg

35. Gurken-Avocado-Suppe

Zubereitungszeit: 10 Minuten | Kochzeit: 0 Minuten | Portionen: 2

Schwierigkeiten: Einfach

Zutaten:

- 1 große Gurke, geschält und gewürfelt
- 1 reife Avocado
- 1 Knoblauchzehe
- 1 Handvoll frischer Dill
- 2 EL Zitronensaft
- 200 ml Wasser
- Salz und Pfeffer nach Geschmack

Zubereitung:

1. Gurke, Avocado, Knoblauch, Dill, Zitronensaft und Wasser in einen Mixer geben.
2. Zu einer glatten Suppe pürieren.
3. Mit Salz und Pfeffer abschmecken.
4. Gekühlt servieren.

Nährwerte (pro Portion): Kalorien: 180 | Fett: 12g | Kohlenhydrate: 15g | Protein: 3g | Zucker: 5g | Natrium: 40mg

36. Rote-Bete-Carpaccio mit Walnüssen

Zubereitungszeit: 15 Minuten | Kochzeit: 0 Minuten | Portionen: 2

Schwierigkeiten: Einfach

Zutaten:

- 2 gekochte Rote Bete, dünn geschnitten
- 50 g Walnüsse, gehackt
- 50 g Rucola
- 2 EL Balsamico-Essig
- 1 EL Olivenöl (nicht erhitzt)
- Salz und Pfeffer nach Geschmack

Zubereitung:

1. Die dünn geschnittene Rote Bete auf zwei Tellern anrichten.
2. Rucola darüber verteilen und mit gehackten Walnüssen bestreuen.
3. Balsamico-Essig und Olivenöl darüber träufeln.
4. Mit Salz und Pfeffer abschmecken und sofort servieren.

Nährwerte (pro Portion): Kalorien: 220 | Fett: 14g | Kohlenhydrate: 18g | Protein: 4g | Zucker: 10g | Natrium: 60mg

37. Gebackener Tofu mit Sesam und Frühlingszwiebeln

Zubereitungszeit: 15 Minuten | Kochzeit: 30 Minuten | Portionen: 2

Schwierigkeiten: Mittel

Zutaten:

- 200 g Tofu, in Würfel geschnitten
- 2 EL Sojasauce (natriumarm)
- 1 EL Sesamöl (nicht erhitzt)
- 1 EL Sesamsamen
- 2 Frühlingszwiebeln, in Ringe geschnitten
- 1 TL Ahornsirup
- 1 TL Ingwer, gerieben
- Salz und Pfeffer nach Geschmack

Zubereitung:

1. Den Tofu in einer Schüssel mit Sojasauce, Sesamöl, Ahornsirup, Ingwer, Salz und Pfeffer marinieren und 15 Minuten ziehen lassen.
2. Den Ofen auf 200 Grad vorheizen.
3. Den Tofu auf ein Backblech legen und 25-30 Minuten backen, bis er goldbraun und knusprig ist.
4. Mit Sesamsamen und Frühlingszwiebeln bestreuen und servieren.

Nährwerte (pro Portion): Kalorien: 250 | Fett: 15g | Kohlenhydrate: 12g | Protein: 16g | Zucker: 4g | Natrium: 300mg

38. Spinat-Salat mit Granatapfel und Mandeln

Zubereitungszeit: 10 Minuten | Kochzeit: 0 Minuten | Portionen: 2

Schwierigkeiten: Einfach

Zutaten:

- 100 g frischer Spinat
- 1 Granatapfel, entkernt
- 1 Avocado, in Scheiben geschnitten
- 50 g Mandeln, gehackt
- 2 EL Zitronensaft
- 1 EL Olivenöl (nicht erhitzt)
- Salz und Pfeffer nach Geschmack

Zubereitung:

1. Den Spinat in eine große Schüssel geben.
2. Granatapfelkerne, Avocado und Mandeln hinzufügen.
3. Zitronensaft und Olivenöl darüber träufeln und mit Salz und Pfeffer abschmecken.
4. Alles gut vermischen und sofort servieren.

Nährwerte (pro Portion): Kalorien: 240 | Fett: 16g | Kohlenhydrate: 22g | Protein: 6g | Zucker: 10g | Natrium: 40mg

39. Linsensalat mit Mango und Avocado

Zubereitungszeit: 15 Minuten | Kochzeit: 20 Minuten | Portionen: 2

Schwierigkeiten: Mittel

Zutaten:

- 150 g grüne Linsen
- 1 reife Mango, gewürfelt
- 1 Avocado, gewürfelt
- 1 kleine rote Zwiebel, fein gehackt
- 1 Handvoll frische Korianderblätter, gehackt
- 2 EL Limettensaft
- 1 EL Olivenöl (nicht erhitzt)
- Salz und Pfeffer nach Geschmack

Zubereitung:

1. Die Linsen in einem Topf mit Wasser zum Kochen bringen und 20 Minuten köcheln lassen, bis sie weich sind. Abgießen und abkühlen lassen.
2. In einer großen Schüssel die abgekühlten Linsen, Mango, Avocado, Zwiebel und Koriander vermischen.
3. Limettensaft und Olivenöl hinzufügen und gut vermischen.
4. Mit Salz und Pfeffer abschmecken und servieren.

Nährwerte (pro Portion): Kalorien: 310 | Fett: 14g | Kohlenhydrate: 40g | Protein: 10g | Zucker: 12g | Natrium: 50mg

40. Auberginen-Röllchen mit Spinat und Pinienkernen

Zubereitungszeit: 20 Minuten | Kochzeit: 30 Minuten | Portionen: 2

Schwierigkeiten: Mittel

Zutaten:

- 1 große Aubergine, längs in dünne Scheiben geschnitten
- 100 g frischer Spinat
- 50 g Pinienkerne, geröstet
- 2 Knoblauchzehen, gehackt
- 1 EL Zitronensaft
- 1 EL Olivenöl (nicht erhitzt)
- Salz und Pfeffer nach Geschmack

Zubereitung:

1. Den Ofen auf 200 Grad vorheizen.
2. Die Auberginenscheiben mit Salz bestreuen und 10 Minuten ziehen lassen, um überschüssige Flüssigkeit zu entfernen. Dann abspülen und trocken tupfen.
3. Die Auberginenscheiben auf ein Backblech legen und 15 Minuten backen, bis sie weich sind.
4. In einer Pfanne den gehackten Knoblauch anbraten, den Spinat hinzufügen und unter Rühren kochen, bis er zusammenfällt.
5. Den Spinat mit Pinienkernen, Zitronensaft, Salz und Pfeffer vermischen.
6. Jeweils einen Löffel der Spinatmischung auf eine Auberginenscheibe geben, aufrollen und die Röllchen auf ein Backblech legen. Weitere 10 Minuten backen.

Nährwerte (pro Portion): Kalorien: 230 | Fett: 14g | Kohlenhydrate: 20g | Protein: 5g | Zucker: 8g | Natrium: 60mg

Kapitel 5: Rezepte für das Abendessen

Entspannende Abendgerichte

41. Gebackener Lachs mit Gemüse

Zubereitungszeit: 10 Minuten | Kochzeit: 25 Minuten | Portionen: 2

Schwierigkeiten: Einfach

Zutaten:

- 2 Lachsfilets (je 150 g)
- 1 Zucchini, in Scheiben geschnitten
- 1 rote Paprika, in Streifen geschnitten
- 1 Karotte, in Scheiben geschnitten
- 1 Zitrone, in Scheiben geschnitten
- 2 EL Olivenöl (nicht erhitzt)
- 1 TL Thymian
- Salz und Pfeffer nach Geschmack

Zubereitung:

1. Den Ofen auf 200 Grad vorheizen.
2. Das Gemüse in eine Auflaufform geben und mit 1 EL Olivenöl, Thymian, Salz und Pfeffer vermischen.
3. Die Lachsfilets auf das Gemüse legen und mit Zitronenscheiben belegen.
4. Mit dem restlichen Olivenöl beträufeln.
5. Im Ofen 25 Minuten backen, bis der Lachs durchgegart ist.

Nährwerte (pro Portion): Kalorien: 350 | Fett: 20g | Kohlenhydrate: 10g | Protein: 30g | Zucker: 5g | Natrium: 150mg

42. Quinoa-Bowl mit gebratenem Gemüse und Tahini-Sauce

Zubereitungszeit: 15 Minuten | Kochzeit: 20 Minuten | Portionen: 2

Schwierigkeiten: Mittel

Zutaten:

- 100 g Quinoa
- 200 ml Wasser
- 1 kleine Aubergine, gewürfelt
- 1 Zucchini, gewürfelt
- 1 rote Paprika, gewürfelt
- 2 EL Olivenöl (nicht erhitzt)
- 2 EL Tahini
- 1 EL Zitronensaft
- 1 Knoblauchzehe, gehackt
- Salz und Pfeffer nach Geschmack

Zubereitung:

1. Die Quinoa in einem Sieb abspülen und mit Wasser in einem Topf zum Kochen bringen. 15 Minuten köcheln lassen, bis die Quinoa weich ist.
2. In einer Pfanne die Aubergine, Zucchini und Paprika bei mittlerer Hitze anbraten, bis das Gemüse weich ist.
3. Das gebratene Gemüse zur gekochten Quinoa geben und gut vermischen.
4. In einer kleinen Schüssel Tahini, Zitronensaft, gehackten Knoblauch, Salz und Pfeffer mit etwas Wasser zu einer glatten Sauce verrühren.
5. Die Quinoa-Gemüse-Mischung in Schalen füllen und mit der Tahini-Sauce servieren.

Nährwerte (pro Portion): Kalorien: 400 | Fett: 18g | Kohlenhydrate: 45g | Protein: 12g | Zucker: 7g | Natrium: 100mg

43. Gefüllte Champignons mit Spinat und Kichererbsen

Zubereitungszeit: 15 Minuten | Kochzeit: 20 Minuten | Portionen: 2

Schwierigkeiten: Mittel

Zutaten:

- 8 große Champignons, Stiele entfernt
- 150 g frischer Spinat

- 1 Dose Kichererbsen (400 g), abgetropft und gespült
- 2 Knoblauchzehen, gehackt
- 1 Zwiebel, gehackt
- 2 EL Olivenöl (nicht erhitzt)
- 1 TL Kreuzkümmel
- Salz und Pfeffer nach Geschmack

Zubereitung:

1. Den Ofen auf 180 Grad vorheizen.
2. In einer Pfanne die gehackte Zwiebel und Knoblauch bei mittlerer Hitze anbraten, bis sie weich sind.
3. Den Spinat hinzufügen und unter Rühren kochen, bis er zusammenfällt.
4. Die abgetropften Kichererbsen und Kreuzkümmel hinzufügen und gut vermischen.
5. Die Champignons mit der Spinat-Kichererbsen-Mischung füllen und 20 Minuten im Ofen backen.

Nährwerte (pro Portion): Kalorien: 280 | Fett: 12g | Kohlenhydrate: 30g | Protein: 10g | Zucker: 5g | Natrium: 150mg

44. Ofen-Gemüse mit Rosmarin

Zubereitungszeit: 10 Minuten | Kochzeit: 30 Minuten | Portionen: 2

Schwierigkeiten: Einfach

Zutaten:

- 2 Karotten, in Stifte geschnitten
- 1 rote Paprika, in Streifen geschnitten
- 1 Süßkartoffel, gewürfelt
- 1 Zucchini, in Scheiben geschnitten
- 2 EL Olivenöl (nicht erhitzt)
- 1 TL Rosmarin
- Salz und Pfeffer nach Geschmack

Zubereitung:

1. Den Ofen auf 200 Grad vorheizen.
2. Das Gemüse in einer großen Schüssel mit Olivenöl, Rosmarin, Salz und Pfeffer vermischen.
3. Das gewürzte Gemüse auf ein Backblech legen.

4. 30 Minuten im Ofen backen, bis das Gemüse weich und goldbraun ist.
5. Sofort servieren.

Nährwerte (pro Portion): Kalorien: 240 | Fett: 12g | Kohlenhydrate: 30g | Protein: 4g | Zucker: 10g | Natrium: 60mg

45. Tomaten-Basilikum-Suppe

Zubereitungszeit: 10 Minuten | Kochzeit: 20 Minuten | Portionen: 2

Schwierigkeiten: Einfach

Zutaten:

- 4 große Tomaten, gehackt
- 1 Zwiebel, gehackt
- 2 Knoblauchzehen, gehackt
- 500 ml Gemüsebrühe
- 1 Handvoll frisches Basilikum, gehackt
- 2 EL Olivenöl (nicht erhitzt)
- Salz und Pfeffer nach Geschmack

Zubereitung:

1. In einem großen Topf die gehackte Zwiebel und Knoblauch bei mittlerer Hitze anbraten, bis sie weich sind.
2. Die gehackten Tomaten hinzufügen und 10 Minuten köcheln lassen.
3. Die Gemüsebrühe einrühren und weitere 10 Minuten kochen lassen.
4. Die Suppe vom Herd nehmen und das gehackte Basilikum hinzufügen.
5. Mit Salz und Pfeffer abschmecken und servieren.

Nährwerte (pro Portion): Kalorien: 180 | Fett: 10g | Kohlenhydrate: 20g | Protein: 4g | Zucker: 10g | Natrium: 150mg

46. Gebackene Aubergine mit Knoblauch-Joghurt-Sauce

Zubereitungszeit: 10 Minuten | Kochzeit: 35 Minuten | Portionen: 2

Schwierigkeiten: Mittel

Zutaten:

- 1 große Aubergine, in Scheiben geschnitten
- 2 EL Olivenöl (nicht erhitzt)
- 200 g griechischer Joghurt
- 2 Knoblauchzehen, gehackt
- 1 EL Zitronensaft
- Salz und Pfeffer nach Geschmack
- 1 Handvoll frische Minze, gehackt

Zubereitung:

1. Den Ofen auf 200 Grad vorheizen.
2. Die Auberginenscheiben mit Olivenöl bestreichen und auf ein Backblech legen.
3. 35 Minuten backen, bis sie weich und goldbraun sind.
4. In einer Schüssel den griechischen Joghurt mit gehacktem Knoblauch, Zitronensaft, Salz und Pfeffer vermischen.
5. Die gebackenen Auberginenscheiben mit der Knoblauch-Joghurt-Sauce und gehackter Minze servieren.

Nährwerte (pro Portion): Kalorien: 220 | Fett: 14g | Kohlenhydrate: 18g | Protein: 6g | Zucker: 8g | Natrium: 100mg

47. Kichererbsen-Curry mit Kokosmilch

Zubereitungszeit: 10 Minuten | Kochzeit: 25 Minuten | Portionen: 2

Schwierigkeiten: Mittel

Zutaten:

- 1 Dose Kichererbsen (400 g), abgetropft und gespült
- 1 Zwiebel, gehackt
- 2 Knoblauchzehen, gehackt
- 1 Stück Ingwer (ca. 2 cm), gerieben
- 1 Dose Kokosmilch (400 ml)
- 2 EL Tomatenmark

- 1 TL Kurkuma
- 1 TL Kreuzkümmel
- 1 TL Koriander
- Salz und Pfeffer nach Geschmack

Zubereitung:

1. In einem großen Topf die gehackte Zwiebel, Knoblauch und geriebenen Ingwer bei mittlerer Hitze anbraten, bis die Zwiebel weich ist.
2. Kurkuma, Kreuzkümmel und Koriander hinzufügen und kurz mit anrösten.
3. Tomatenmark und Kichererbsen hinzufügen und gut vermischen.
4. Kokosmilch einrühren und das Curry bei niedriger Hitze etwa 20 Minuten köcheln lassen.
5. Mit Salz und Pfeffer abschmecken und servieren.

Nährwerte (pro Portion): Kalorien: 320 | Fett: 18g | Kohlenhydrate: 28g | Protein: 8g | Zucker: 6g | Natrium: 150mg

48. Spaghetti aus Zucchini mit Tomaten und Basilikum

Zubereitungszeit: 10 Minuten | Kochzeit: 10 Minuten | Portionen: 2

Schwierigkeiten: Einfach

Zutaten:

- 2 große Zucchini, spiralförmig geschnitten
- 200 g Kirschtomaten, halbiert
- 2 Knoblauchzehen, gehackt
- 1 Handvoll frisches Basilikum, gehackt
- 2 EL Olivenöl (nicht erhitzt)
- Salz und Pfeffer nach Geschmack

Zubereitung:

1. Die Zucchini-Spaghetti mit etwas Salz bestreuen und 10 Minuten ziehen lassen, um überschüssige Feuchtigkeit zu entfernen.
2. In einer großen Pfanne die gehackten Knoblauchzehen bei mittlerer Hitze anbraten, bis sie duften.
3. Die Kirschtomaten hinzufügen und 5 Minuten köcheln lassen, bis sie weich sind.
4. Die abgetropften Zucchini-Spaghetti hinzufügen und kurz erhitzen.
5. Mit Basilikum, Salz und Pfeffer abschmecken und servieren.

Nährwerte (pro Portion): Kalorien: 180 | Fett: 10g | Kohlenhydrate: 15g | Protein: 4g | Zucker: 8g | Natrium: 50mg

49. Linseneintopf mit Gemüse

Zubereitungszeit: 10 Minuten | Kochzeit: 30 Minuten | Portionen: 2
Schwierigkeiten: Mittel
Zutaten:

- 150 g grüne Linsen
- 1 Zwiebel, gehackt
- 2 Karotten, gewürfelt
- 1 Selleriestange, gewürfelt
- 2 Knoblauchzehen, gehackt
- 1 Liter Gemüsebrühe
- 1 TL Thymian
- 1 TL Kreuzkümmel
- Salz und Pfeffer nach Geschmack
- 1 Handvoll frische Petersilie, gehackt

Zubereitung:

1. In einem großen Topf die gehackte Zwiebel, Karotten, Sellerie und Knoblauch bei mittlerer Hitze anbraten, bis das Gemüse weich ist.
2. Thymian und Kreuzkümmel hinzufügen und kurz mit anrösten.
3. Die Linsen und Gemüsebrühe hinzufügen und zum Kochen bringen.
4. Die Hitze reduzieren und den Eintopf 25-30 Minuten köcheln lassen, bis die Linsen weich sind.
5. Mit Salz und Pfeffer abschmecken, Petersilie unterrühren und servieren.

Nährwerte (pro Portion): Kalorien: 280 | Fett: 5g | Kohlenhydrate: 45g | Protein: 12g | Zucker: 8g | Natrium: 300mg

50. Gebratene Pilze mit Kräutern

Zubereitungszeit: 10 Minuten | Kochzeit: 20 Minuten | Portionen: 2

Schwierigkeiten: Einfach

Zutaten:

- 300 g gemischte Pilze, in Scheiben geschnitten
- 2 Knoblauchzehen, gehackt
- 1 Zwiebel, gehackt
- 2 EL Olivenöl (nicht erhitzt)
- 1 TL Thymian
- 1 TL Rosmarin
- Salz und Pfeffer nach Geschmack
- 1 Handvoll frische Petersilie, gehackt

Zubereitung:

1. In einer großen Pfanne die gehackten Zwiebel und Knoblauch bei mittlerer Hitze anbraten, bis sie weich sind.
2. Die Pilze hinzufügen und unter Rühren kochen, bis sie weich und goldbraun sind.
3. Thymian und Rosmarin hinzufügen und gut vermischen.
4. Mit Salz und Pfeffer abschmecken und die gehackte Petersilie unterrühren.
5. Sofort servieren.

Nährwerte (pro Portion): Kalorien: 220 | Fett: 14g | Kohlenhydrate: 18g | Protein: 6g | Zucker: 5g | Natrium: 100mg

Hauptgerichte für das Wohlbefinden

51. Linsensalat mit geröstetem Gemüse

Zubereitungszeit: 15 Minuten | Kochzeit: 30 Minuten | Portionen: 2

Schwierigkeiten: Mittel

Zutaten:

- 150 g grüne Linsen
- 1 rote Paprika, in Streifen geschnitten
- 1 Zucchini, in Scheiben geschnitten
- 1 Karotte, in Scheiben geschnitten
- 1 rote Zwiebel, in Ringe geschnitten
- 2 EL Olivenöl (nicht erhitzt)
- 2 EL Balsamico-Essig
- 1 Handvoll frische Petersilie, gehackt
- Salz und Pfeffer nach Geschmack

Zubereitung:

1. Die Linsen in einem Topf mit Wasser zum Kochen bringen und 20 Minuten köcheln lassen, bis sie weich sind. Abgießen und abkühlen lassen.
2. Den Ofen auf 200 Grad vorheizen.
3. Paprika, Zucchini, Karotte und Zwiebel mit 1 EL Olivenöl, Salz und Pfeffer vermischen und auf ein Backblech legen.
4. 30 Minuten im Ofen rösten, bis das Gemüse weich und leicht gebräunt ist.
5. Die Linsen und das geröstete Gemüse in einer Schüssel vermischen, mit Balsamico-Essig und dem restlichen Olivenöl beträufeln und die gehackte Petersilie unterheben.
6. Sofort servieren.

Nährwerte (pro Portion): Kalorien: 350 | Fett: 14g | Kohlenhydrate: 45g | Protein: 12g | Zucker: 10g | Natrium: 150mg

52. Blumenkohl-Curry mit Kokosmilch

Zubereitungszeit: 15 Minuten | Kochzeit: 25 Minuten | Portionen: 2

Schwierigkeiten: Mittel

Zutaten:

- 1 kleiner Blumenkohl, in Röschen zerteilt
- 1 Zwiebel, gehackt
- 2 Knoblauchzehen, gehackt
- 1 Stück Ingwer (ca. 2 cm), gerieben
- 1 Dose Kokosmilch (400 ml)
- 1 Dose Tomaten (400 g)
- 1 TL Kurkuma
- 1 TL Kreuzkümmel
- 1 TL Koriander
- Salz und Pfeffer nach Geschmack
- 1 Handvoll frische Korianderblätter, gehackt

Zubereitung:

1. In einem großen Topf die gehackte Zwiebel, Knoblauch und geriebenen Ingwer bei mittlerer Hitze anbraten, bis die Zwiebel weich ist.
2. Kurkuma, Kreuzkümmel und Koriander hinzufügen und kurz mit anrösten.
3. Blumenkohlröschen, Kokosmilch und Tomaten hinzufügen und gut vermischen.
4. Das Curry bei niedriger Hitze etwa 20 Minuten köcheln lassen, bis der Blumenkohl weich ist.
5. Mit Salz und Pfeffer abschmecken, gehackte Korianderblätter unterrühren und servieren.

Nährwerte (pro Portion): Kalorien: 300 | Fett: 18g | Kohlenhydrate: 28g | Protein: 6g | Zucker: 10g | Natrium: 200mg

53. Zucchini-Lasagne mit Spinat

Zubereitungszeit: 20 Minuten | Kochzeit: 40 Minuten | Portionen: 2

Schwierigkeiten: Mittel

Zutaten:

- 2 große Zucchini, längs in dünne Scheiben geschnitten
- 200 g frischer Spinat

- 1 Zwiebel, gehackt
- 2 Knoblauchzehen, gehackt
- 1 Dose Tomaten (400 g)
- 200 g Ricotta
- 1 Ei
- 1 TL Oregano
- 1 TL Basilikum
- Salz und Pfeffer nach Geschmack
- 50 g geriebener Parmesan

Zubereitung:

1. Den Ofen auf 180 Grad vorheizen.
2. In einer Pfanne die gehackte Zwiebel und Knoblauch bei mittlerer Hitze anbraten, bis sie weich sind.
3. Den Spinat hinzufügen und unter Rühren kochen, bis er zusammenfällt. Tomaten, Oregano und Basilikum hinzufügen und gut vermischen.
4. In einer Schüssel Ricotta und Ei verquirlen und mit Salz und Pfeffer abschmecken.
5. Eine Schicht Zucchinischeiben in eine Auflaufform legen, die Ricottamischung und dann die Spinat-Tomaten-Mischung darüber verteilen. Diesen Vorgang wiederholen, bis alle Zutaten aufgebraucht sind.
6. Mit geriebenem Parmesan bestreuen und 40 Minuten backen, bis die Lasagne goldbraun und sprudelnd ist.

Nährwerte (pro Portion): Kalorien: 400 | Fett: 22g | Kohlenhydrate: 28g | Protein: 20g | Zucker: 10g | Natrium: 300mg

54. Kichererbsen-Bowl mit gebratenem Gemüse

Zubereitungszeit: 15 Minuten | Kochzeit: 25 Minuten | Portionen: 2

Schwierigkeiten: Mittel

Zutaten:

- 1 Dose Kichererbsen (400 g), abgetropft und gespült
- 1 rote Paprika, in Streifen geschnitten
- 1 Zucchini, gewürfelt
- 1 Karotte, in Scheiben geschnitten
- 1 Zwiebel, gehackt

- 2 EL Olivenöl (nicht erhitzt)
- 1 TL Kreuzkümmel
- 1 TL Paprika
- Salz und Pfeffer nach Geschmack
- 1 Handvoll frische Petersilie, gehackt
- 1 EL Zitronensaft

Zubereitung:

1. Den Ofen auf 200 Grad vorheizen.
2. Paprika, Zucchini, Karotte und Zwiebel mit 1 EL Olivenöl, Kreuzkümmel, Paprika, Salz und Pfeffer vermischen und auf ein Backblech legen.
3. 25 Minuten im Ofen rösten, bis das Gemüse weich und leicht gebräunt ist.
4. Die gerösteten Kichererbsen in einer Pfanne mit 1 EL Olivenöl bei mittlerer Hitze anbraten, bis sie knusprig sind.
5. Das geröstete Gemüse und die Kichererbsen in Schalen füllen, mit gehackter Petersilie und Zitronensaft bestreuen und servieren.

Nährwerte (pro Portion): Kalorien: 350 | Fett: 14g | Kohlenhydrate: 45g | Protein: 10g | Zucker: 10g | Natrium: 200mg

55. Gebratener Tofu mit Sesam und Brokkoli

Zubereitungszeit: 15 Minuten | Kochzeit: 20 Minuten | Portionen: 2

Schwierigkeiten: Mittel

Zutaten:

- 200 g Tofu, in Würfel geschnitten
- 1 Kopf Brokkoli, in Röschen zerteilt
- 1 rote Paprika, in Streifen geschnitten
- 2 Knoblauchzehen, gehackt
- 1 TL Ingwer, gerieben
- 2 EL Sojasauce (natriumarm)
- 1 EL Sesamöl (nicht erhitzt)
- 1 EL Sesamsamen
- Salz und Pfeffer nach Geschmack

Zubereitung:

1. Den Tofu in einer Pfanne mit 1 EL Sesamöl bei mittlerer Hitze anbraten, bis er goldbraun

und knusprig ist. Aus der Pfanne nehmen und beiseite stellen.

2. In derselben Pfanne den gehackten Knoblauch und geriebenen Ingwer anbraten, bis sie duften.
3. Brokkoli und Paprika hinzufügen und unter Rühren kochen, bis das Gemüse weich ist.
4. Den gebratenen Tofu zurück in die Pfanne geben und mit Sojasauce, Sesamsamen, Salz und Pfeffer abschmecken.
5. Sofort servieren.

Nährwerte (pro Portion): Kalorien: 300 | Fett: 16g | Kohlenhydrate: 20g | Protein: 20g | Zucker: 6g | Natrium: 400mg

56. Quinoa-Salat mit Avocado und Mango

Zubereitungszeit: 15 Minuten | Kochzeit: 15 Minuten | Portionen: 2

Schwierigkeiten: Einfach

Zutaten:

- 100 g Quinoa
- 200 ml Wasser
- 1 reife Mango, gewürfelt
- 1 Avocado, gewürfelt
- 1 rote Paprika, gewürfelt
- 1 kleine rote Zwiebel, fein gehackt
- 1 Handvoll frische Korianderblätter, gehackt
- 2 EL Limettensaft
- 1 EL Olivenöl (nicht erhitzt)
- Salz und Pfeffer nach Geschmack

Zubereitung:

1. Die Quinoa in einem Sieb abspülen und mit Wasser in einem Topf zum Kochen bringen. 15 Minuten köcheln lassen, bis die Quinoa weich ist und die Flüssigkeit absorbiert wurde. Abkühlen lassen.
2. In einer großen Schüssel die abgekühlte Quinoa, Mango, Avocado, Paprika, Zwiebel und Koriander vermischen.
3. Limettensaft und Olivenöl hinzufügen und gut vermischen.
4. Mit Salz und Pfeffer abschmecken und servieren.

Nährwerte (pro Portion): Kalorien: 350 | Fett: 18g | Kohlenhydrate: 40g | Protein: 8g | Zucker: 12g | Natrium: 100mg

57. Gebackene Süßkartoffeln mit Tahini-Dressing

Zubereitungszeit: 10 Minuten | Kochzeit: 40 Minuten | Portionen: 2

Schwierigkeiten: Einfach

Zutaten:

- 2 große Süßkartoffeln
- 2 EL Tahini
- 1 EL Zitronensaft
- 1 Knoblauchzehe, gehackt
- 2 EL Wasser
- 1 TL Kreuzkümmel
- Salz und Pfeffer nach Geschmack
- 1 Handvoll frische Petersilie, gehackt

Zubereitung:

1. Den Ofen auf 200 Grad vorheizen.
2. Die Süßkartoffeln waschen, trocknen und mit einer Gabel ein paar Mal einstechen. Auf ein Backblech legen und 40 Minuten backen, bis sie weich sind.
3. Während die Süßkartoffeln backen, Tahini, Zitronensaft, gehackten Knoblauch, Wasser, Kreuzkümmel, Salz und Pfeffer in einer Schüssel zu einer glatten Sauce verrühren.
4. Die gebackenen Süßkartoffeln längs aufschneiden und mit dem Tahini-Dressing und gehackter Petersilie servieren.

Nährwerte (pro Portion): Kalorien: 300 | Fett: 10g | Kohlenhydrate: 50g | Protein: 5g | Zucker: 10g | Natrium: 60mg

58. Spinat-Curry mit Kichererbsen

Zubereitungszeit: 15 Minuten | Kochzeit: 20 Minuten | Portionen: 2

Schwierigkeiten: Mittel

Zutaten:

- 200 g frischer Spinat
- 1 Dose Kichererbsen (400 g), abgetropft und gespült
- 1 Zwiebel, gehackt
- 2 Knoblauchzehen, gehackt
- 1 Stück Ingwer (ca. 2 cm), gerieben
- 1 Dose Kokosmilch (400 ml)
- 1 Dose Tomaten (400 g)
- 1 TL Kurkuma
- 1 TL Kreuzkümmel
- 1 TL Koriander
- Salz und Pfeffer nach Geschmack

Zubereitung:

1. In einem großen Topf die gehackte Zwiebel, Knoblauch und geriebenen Ingwer bei mittlerer Hitze anbraten, bis die Zwiebel weich ist.
2. Kurkuma, Kreuzkümmel und Koriander hinzufügen und kurz mit anrösten.
3. Spinat, Kichererbsen, Kokosmilch und Tomaten hinzufügen und gut vermischen.
4. Das Curry bei niedriger Hitze etwa 20 Minuten köcheln lassen, bis der Spinat zusammengefallen und die Aromen gut durchgezogen sind.
5. Mit Salz und Pfeffer abschmecken und servieren.

Nährwerte (pro Portion): Kalorien: 350 | Fett: 18g | Kohlenhydrate: 35g | Protein: 10g | Zucker: 8g | Natrium: 150mg

59. Gebackene Aubergine mit Tomaten und Basilikum

Zubereitungszeit: 10 Minuten | Kochzeit: 30 Minuten | Portionen: 2

Schwierigkeiten: Mittel

Zutaten:

- 2 große Auberginen, längs halbiert
- 2 Tomaten, gewürfelt

- 2 Knoblauchzehen, gehackt
- 1 Handvoll frisches Basilikum, gehackt
- 2 EL Olivenöl (nicht erhitzt)
- Salz und Pfeffer nach Geschmack

Zubereitung:

1. Den Ofen auf 200 Grad vorheizen.
2. Die Auberginenhälften mit einem Messer einritzen und mit 1 EL Olivenöl bestreichen. Auf ein Backblech legen und 30 Minuten backen, bis sie weich sind.
3. In einer Pfanne die gehackten Knoblauchzehen anbraten, bis sie duften. Die gewürfelten Tomaten hinzufügen und 5 Minuten köcheln lassen.
4. Die gebackenen Auberginenhälften mit der Tomaten-Knoblauch-Mischung belegen und mit gehacktem Basilikum bestreuen.
5. Mit Salz und Pfeffer abschmecken und servieren.

Nährwerte (pro Portion): Kalorien: 250 | Fett: 14g | Kohlenhydrate: 25g | Protein: 4g | Zucker: 10g | Natrium: 50mg

60. Karotten-Ingwer-Suppe

Zubereitungszeit: 10 Minuten | Kochzeit: 20 Minuten | Portionen: 2

Schwierigkeiten: Einfach

Zutaten:

- 500 g Karotten, geschält und in Scheiben geschnitten
- 1 Zwiebel, gehackt
- 2 Knoblauchzehen, gehackt
- 1 Stück Ingwer (ca. 2 cm), gerieben
- 750 ml Gemüsebrühe
- 1 TL Kurkuma
- 1 EL Olivenöl (nicht erhitzt)
- Salz und Pfeffer nach Geschmack
- 1 Handvoll frische Petersilie, gehackt

Zubereitung:

1. In einem großen Topf die gehackte Zwiebel, Knoblauch und geriebenen Ingwer bei mittlerer Hitze anbraten, bis die Zwiebel weich ist.
2. Karottenscheiben und Kurkuma hinzufügen und gut vermischen.

3. Die Gemüsebrühe einrühren und die Suppe zum Kochen bringen. 20 Minuten köcheln lassen, bis die Karotten weich sind.
4. Die Suppe pürieren, bis sie glatt ist, und mit Salz und Pfeffer abschmecken.
5. Mit gehackter Petersilie bestreuen und servieren.

Nährwerte (pro Portion): Kalorien: 220 | Fett: 8g | Kohlenhydrate: 30g | Protein: 4g | Zucker: 15g | Natrium: 200mg

Kapitel 6: Süßes

Süße Gerichte ohne Entzündungsförderer

61. Avocado-Schokoladenmousse

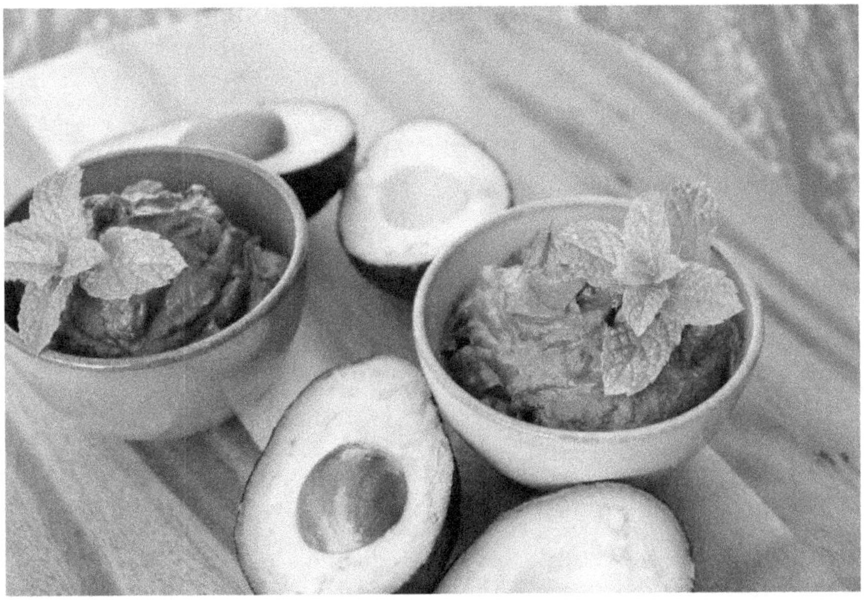

Zubereitungszeit: 10 Minuten | Kochzeit: 0 Minuten | Portionen: 2

Schwierigkeiten: Einfach

Zutaten:

- 2 reife Avocados
- 3 EL ungesüßtes Kakaopulver
- 2 EL Ahornsirup
- 1 TL Vanilleextrakt
- Eine Prise Salz
- Frische Beeren zum Garnieren

Zubereitung:

1. Die Avocados schälen und entkernen.
2. Das Avocado-Fruchtfleisch zusammen mit Kakaopulver, Ahornsirup, Vanilleextrakt und Salz in einen Mixer geben.

3. Zu einer glatten Masse pürieren.
4. Die Mousse in Dessertschalen füllen und mindestens 30 Minuten im Kühlschrank kühlen.
5. Mit frischen Beeren garnieren und servieren.

Nährwerte (pro Portion): Kalorien: 250 | Fett: 18g | Kohlenhydrate: 25g | Protein: 3g | Zucker: 10g | Natrium: 50mg

62. Gebackene Äpfel mit Walnüssen und Zimt

Zubereitungszeit: 10 Minuten | Kochzeit: 25 Minuten | Portionen: 2

Schwierigkeiten: Einfach

Zutaten:

- 2 große Äpfel
- 2 EL gehackte Walnüsse
- 1 EL Rosinen
- 1 TL Zimt
- 1 EL Ahornsirup
- 1 TL Kokosöl

Zubereitung:

1. Den Ofen auf 180 Grad vorheizen.
2. Die Äpfel waschen und das Kerngehäuse entfernen.
3. Walnüsse, Rosinen, Zimt und Ahornsirup in einer kleinen Schüssel vermischen.
4. Die Mischung in die Äpfel füllen.
5. Die Äpfel in eine Auflaufform setzen und mit Kokosöl bestreichen.
6. 25 Minuten im Ofen backen, bis die Äpfel weich sind.

Nährwerte (pro Portion): Kalorien: 180 | Fett: 8g | Kohlenhydrate: 30g | Protein: 2g | Zucker: 20g | Natrium: 10mg

63. Himbeer-Kokos-Energiebällchen

Zubereitungszeit: 15 Minuten | Kochzeit: 0 Minuten | Portionen: 2

Schwierigkeiten: Einfach

Zutaten:

- 100 g getrocknete Himbeeren
- 50 g Mandeln
- 50 g Kokosflocken
- 2 EL Ahornsirup
- 1 TL Vanilleextrakt

Zubereitung:

1. Die getrockneten Himbeeren, Mandeln und Kokosflocken in einen Mixer geben und fein zerkleinern.
2. Ahornsirup und Vanilleextrakt hinzufügen und zu einer klebrigen Masse vermischen.
3. Aus der Masse kleine Bällchen formen.
4. Die Energiebällchen in Kokosflocken wälzen.
5. Im Kühlschrank aufbewahren und nach Bedarf genießen.

Nährwerte (pro Portion): Kalorien: 250 | Fett: 15g | Kohlenhydrate: 25g | Protein: 4g | Zucker: 18g | Natrium: 5mg

64. Bananen-Eiscreme mit Beeren

Zubereitungszeit: 10 Minuten | Kochzeit: 0 Minuten | Portionen: 2

Schwierigkeiten: Einfach

Zutaten:

- 2 reife Bananen, gefroren
- 100 g gemischte Beeren
- 1 TL Vanilleextrakt

Zubereitung:

1. Die gefrorenen Bananen in Stücke schneiden.
2. Die Bananenstücke zusammen mit den Beeren und dem Vanilleextrakt in einen Mixer geben.
3. Zu einer glatten Masse pürieren.
4. Die Eiscreme sofort servieren oder im Gefrierschrank aufbewahren.

Nährwerte (pro Portion): Kalorien: 150 | Fett: 1g | Kohlenhydrate: 35g | Protein: 2g | Zucker: 20g | Natrium: 0mg

65. Quinoa-Pudding mit Zimt und Ahornsirup

Zubereitungszeit: 10 Minuten | Kochzeit: 20 Minuten | Portionen: 2

Schwierigkeiten: Mittel

Zutaten:

- 100 g Quinoa
- 300 ml Mandelmilch
- 1 TL Zimt
- 2 EL Ahornsirup
- 1 TL Vanilleextrakt
- Frische Beeren zum Garnieren

Zubereitung:

1. Die Quinoa in einem Sieb abspülen.
2. Die Mandelmilch in einem Topf zum Kochen bringen, die Quinoa hinzufügen und 15-20 Minuten köcheln lassen, bis die Quinoa weich ist.
3. Zimt, Ahornsirup und Vanilleextrakt unterrühren.
4. Den Pudding in Schalen füllen und mit frischen Beeren garnieren.
5. Warm oder gekühlt servieren.

Nährwerte (pro Portion): Kalorien: 220 | Fett: 5g | Kohlenhydrate: 40g | Protein: 6g | Zucker: 15g | Natrium: 40mg

66. Mandel-Kakao-Energieriegel

Zubereitungszeit: 15 Minuten | Kochzeit: 0 Minuten | Portionen: 2

Schwierigkeiten: Mittel

Zutaten:

- 100 g Mandeln
- 50 g Haferflocken
- 2 EL Kakaopulver
- 3 EL Ahornsirup
- 1 TL Vanilleextrakt

Zubereitung:

1. Die Mandeln und Haferflocken in einem Mixer grob zerkleinern.
2. Kakaopulver, Ahornsirup und Vanilleextrakt hinzufügen und gut vermischen.
3. Die Masse auf ein mit Backpapier ausgelegtes Backblech drücken und gleichmäßig verteilen.
4. Für 1 Stunde im Kühlschrank fest werden lassen.
5. In Riegel schneiden und genießen.

Nährwerte (pro Portion): Kalorien: 250 | Fett: 12g | Kohlenhydrate: 30g | Protein: 6g | Zucker: 15g | Natrium: 10mg

67. Birnenkompott mit Vanille und Ingwer

Zubereitungszeit: 10 Minuten | Kochzeit: 20 Minuten | Portionen: 2

Schwierigkeiten: Einfach

Zutaten:

- 2 reife Birnen, geschält und gewürfelt
- 1 TL frischer Ingwer, gerieben
- 1 TL Vanilleextrakt
- 2 EL Ahornsirup
- 100 ml Wasser

Zubereitung:

1. Die gewürfelten Birnen zusammen mit Ingwer, Vanilleextrakt, Ahornsirup und Wasser in einen Topf geben.
2. Zum Kochen bringen und dann die Hitze reduzieren.
3. 20 Minuten köcheln lassen, bis die Birnen weich sind.
4. Das Kompott in Schalen füllen und warm oder gekühlt servieren.

Nährwerte (pro Portion): Kalorien: 150 | Fett: 0g | Kohlenhydrate: 35g | Protein: 1g | Zucker: 25g | Natrium: 0mg

68. Kokos-Mandel-Kekse

Zubereitungszeit: 15 Minuten | Kochzeit: 15 Minuten | Portionen: 2

Schwierigkeiten: Mittel

Zutaten:

- 100 g Kokosmehl
- 50 g gemahlene Mandeln
- 2 EL Ahornsirup
- 1 TL Vanilleextrakt
- 2 EL Kokosöl, geschmolzen
- 1 Ei

Zubereitung:

1. Den Ofen auf 180 Grad vorheizen und ein Backblech mit Backpapier auslegen.
2. Kokosmehl und gemahlene Mandeln in einer Schüssel vermischen.
3. Ahornsirup, Vanilleextrakt, geschmolzenes Kokosöl und Ei hinzufügen und gut vermischen.
4. Aus der Masse kleine Kugeln formen und auf das Backblech legen.
5. Die Kekse 15 Minuten backen, bis sie goldbraun sind.

Nährwerte (pro Portion): Kalorien: 200 | Fett: 14g | Kohlenhydrate: 15g | Protein: 5g | Zucker: 8g | Natrium: 30mg

69. Chia-Samen-Pudding mit Blaubeeren

Zubereitungszeit: 10 Minuten | Kochzeit: 0 Minuten | Portionen: 2

Schwierigkeiten: Einfach

Zutaten:

- 4 EL Chiasamen
- 250 ml Mandelmilch
- 1 TL Ahornsirup
- 1 TL Vanilleextrakt
- 100 g frische Blaubeeren

Zubereitung:

1. Chiasamen, Mandelmilch, Ahornsirup und Vanilleextrakt in einer Schüssel gut verrühren.
2. Abdecken und über Nacht im Kühlschrank quellen lassen.

3. Vor dem Servieren die Blaubeeren über den Chia-Pudding verteilen.
4. Sofort genießen.

Nährwerte (pro Portion): Kalorien: 220 | Fett: 10g | Kohlenhydrate: 25g | Protein: 4g | Zucker: 10g | Natrium: 20mg

Gesunde Alternativen zu Desserts

70. Mandel-Himbeer-Kugeln

Zubereitungszeit: 15 Minuten | Kochzeit: 0 Minuten | Portionen: 2

Schwierigkeiten: Einfach

Zutaten:

- 100 g Mandeln
- 50 g getrocknete Himbeeren
- 2 EL Kokosöl, geschmolzen
- 2 EL Ahornsirup
- 1 TL Vanilleextrakt

Zubereitung:

1. Die Mandeln und getrockneten Himbeeren in einem Mixer fein zerkleinern.
2. Kokosöl, Ahornsirup und Vanilleextrakt hinzufügen und zu einer klebrigen Masse vermischen.
3. Aus der Masse kleine Kugeln formen.
4. Im Kühlschrank fest werden lassen und nach Bedarf genießen.

Nährwerte (pro Portion): Kalorien: 250 | Fett: 18g | Kohlenhydrate: 20g | Protein: 6g | Zucker: 12g | Natrium: 5mg

71. Gefrorene Bananen-Sandwiches mit Erdnussbutter

Zubereitungszeit: 10 Minuten | Kochzeit: 0 Minuten | Portionen: 2

Schwierigkeiten: Einfach

Zutaten:

- 1 reife Banane
- 2 EL Erdnussbutter (ohne Zuckerzusatz)
- 50 g dunkle Schokolade (mindestens 70% Kakao)

Zubereitung:

1. Die Banane in 1 cm dicke Scheiben schneiden.
2. Jeweils eine Scheibe Banane mit Erdnussbutter bestreichen und eine zweite Scheibe darauflegen, um ein Sandwich zu bilden.

3. Die dunkle Schokolade im Wasserbad schmelzen.
4. Die Bananen-Sandwiches in die geschmolzene Schokolade tauchen und auf ein Backpapier legen.
5. Im Gefrierschrank fest werden lassen und gekühlt servieren.

Nährwerte (pro Portion): Kalorien: 220 | Fett: 12g | Kohlenhydrate: 28g | Protein: 4g | Zucker: 18g | Natrium: 40mg

72. Apfel-Zimt-Crumble

Zubereitungszeit: 15 Minuten | Kochzeit: 25 Minuten | Portionen: 2

Schwierigkeiten: Mittel

Zutaten:

- 2 große Äpfel, geschält und in Scheiben geschnitten
- 1 TL Zimt
- 2 EL Ahornsirup
- 50 g Haferflocken
- 50 g gemahlene Mandeln
- 2 EL Kokosöl, geschmolzen

Zubereitung:

1. Den Ofen auf 180 Grad vorheizen.
2. Die Apfelscheiben in eine Auflaufform geben und mit Zimt und Ahornsirup vermischen.
3. Haferflocken, gemahlene Mandeln und Kokosöl in einer Schüssel vermischen, bis eine krümelige Masse entsteht.
4. Die Hafer-Mandel-Mischung gleichmäßig über die Äpfel streuen.
5. 25 Minuten backen, bis der Crumble goldbraun ist.

Nährwerte (pro Portion): Kalorien: 280 | Fett: 14g | Kohlenhydrate: 35g | Protein: 5g | Zucker: 18g | Natrium: 20mg

73. Avocado-Limetten-Kuchen

Zubereitungszeit: 20 Minuten | Kochzeit: 0 Minuten | Portionen: 2

Schwierigkeiten: Mittel

Zutaten:

- 1 reife Avocado
- 100 g gemahlene Mandeln
- 2 EL Kokosöl, geschmolzen
- 2 EL Ahornsirup
- Saft und Schale von 2 Limetten
- 1 TL Vanilleextrakt

Zubereitung:

1. Die Avocado schälen und entkernen.
2. Avocado, gemahlene Mandeln, Kokosöl, Ahornsirup, Limettensaft, Limettenschale und Vanilleextrakt in einen Mixer geben und zu einer glatten Masse pürieren.
3. Die Masse in eine kleine Kuchenform drücken und im Kühlschrank fest werden lassen.
4. Vor dem Servieren in Stücke schneiden und genießen.

Nährwerte (pro Portion): Kalorien: 280 | Fett: 20g | Kohlenhydrate: 20g | Protein: 5g | Zucker: 12g | Natrium: 10mg

74. Beeren-Quark-Dessert

Zubereitungszeit: 10 Minuten | Kochzeit: 0 Minuten | Portionen: 2

Schwierigkeiten: Einfach

Zutaten:

- 200 g Magerquark
- 100 g gemischte Beeren (frisch oder gefroren)
- 1 TL Honig
- 1 TL Vanilleextrakt
- 1 EL gehackte Mandeln

Zubereitung:

1. Den Magerquark in eine Schüssel geben.
2. Die Beeren über den Quark verteilen.
3. Honig und Vanilleextrakt über die Beeren träufeln.

4. Mit gehackten Mandeln bestreuen und sofort servieren.

Nährwerte (pro Portion): Kalorien: 180 | Fett: 5g | Kohlenhydrate: 20g | Protein: 12g | Zucker: 15g | Natrium: 40mg

75. Kokos-Limetten-Eis

Zubereitungszeit: 15 Minuten | Kochzeit: 0 Minuten | Portionen: 2

Schwierigkeiten: Einfach

Zutaten:

- 200 ml Kokosmilch
- Saft und Schale von 1 Limette
- 2 EL Ahornsirup
- 1 TL Vanilleextrakt

Zubereitung:

1. Kokosmilch, Limettensaft, Limettenschale, Ahornsirup und Vanilleextrakt in einer Schüssel gut vermischen.
2. Die Mischung in eine Eismaschine geben und nach den Anweisungen der Maschine einfrieren.
3. Alternativ die Mischung in eine flache Form gießen und im Gefrierschrank einfrieren, dabei alle 30 Minuten umrühren, bis die gewünschte Konsistenz erreicht ist.
4. Sofort servieren.

Nährwerte (pro Portion): Kalorien: 200 | Fett: 15g | Kohlenhydrate: 18g | Protein: 2g | Zucker: 12g | Natrium: 10mg

76. Chia-Kokos-Pudding mit Ananas

Zubereitungszeit: 10 Minuten | Kochzeit: 0 Minuten | Portionen: 2

Schwierigkeiten: Einfach

Zutaten:

- 4 EL Chiasamen
- 250 ml Kokosmilch
- 1 TL Vanilleextrakt
- 1 EL Ahornsirup
- 100 g frische Ananas, gewürfelt

Zubereitung:

1. Chiasamen, Kokosmilch, Vanilleextrakt und Ahornsirup in einer Schüssel gut verrühren.
2. Abdecken und über Nacht im Kühlschrank quellen lassen.
3. Vor dem Servieren die gewürfelte Ananas über den Chia-Pudding verteilen.
4. Sofort genießen.

Nährwerte (pro Portion): Kalorien: 220 | Fett: 12g | Kohlenhydrate: 25g | Protein: 4g | Zucker: 15g | Natrium: 20mg

77. Geröstete Pfirsiche mit Joghurt und Honig

Zubereitungszeit: 10 Minuten | Kochzeit: 20 Minuten | Portionen: 2

Schwierigkeiten: Einfach

Zutaten:

- 2 reife Pfirsiche, halbiert und entkernt
- 200 g griechischer Joghurt
- 1 EL Honig
- 1 TL Zimt
- 1 EL gehackte Pistazien

Zubereitung:

1. Den Ofen auf 180 Grad vorheizen.
2. Die Pfirsichhälften auf ein Backblech legen und mit Zimt bestreuen.
3. 20 Minuten im Ofen rösten, bis sie weich und leicht gebräunt sind.
4. Die gerösteten Pfirsiche mit griechischem Joghurt und Honig servieren.
5. Mit gehackten Pistazien bestreuen und genießen.

Nährwerte (pro Portion): Kalorien: 210 | Fett: 7g | Kohlenhydrate: 28g | Protein: 8g | Zucker: 20g | Natrium: 40mg

78. Matcha-Kokos-Energieballs

Zubereitungszeit: 15 Minuten | Kochzeit: 0 Minuten | Portionen: 2

Schwierigkeiten: Einfach

Zutaten:

- 100 g Mandeln
- 50 g Kokosflocken
- 1 TL Matcha-Pulver
- 2 EL Ahornsirup
- 1 TL Vanilleextrakt

Zubereitung:

1. Die Mandeln und Kokosflocken in einem Mixer fein zerkleinern.
2. Matcha-Pulver, Ahornsirup und Vanilleextrakt hinzufügen und gut vermischen.
3. Aus der Masse kleine Kugeln formen.
4. Im Kühlschrank fest werden lassen und nach Bedarf genießen.

Nährwerte (pro Portion): Kalorien: 250 | Fett: 15g | Kohlenhydrate: 20g | Protein: 6g | Zucker: 12g | Natrium: 5mg

79. Heidelbeer-Kokos-Smoothie

Zubereitungszeit: 5 Minuten | Kochzeit: 0 Minuten | Portionen: 2

Schwierigkeiten: Einfach

Zutaten:

- 200 g frische Heidelbeeren
- 200 ml Kokosmilch
- 1 Banane
- 1 TL Ahornsirup
- 1 TL Vanilleextrakt

Zubereitung:

1. Die Heidelbeeren, Kokosmilch, Banane, Ahornsirup und Vanilleextrakt in einen Mixer geben.

2. Zu einem glatten Smoothie pürieren.
3. In Gläser füllen und sofort genießen.

Nährwerte (pro Portion): Kalorien: 180 | Fett: 8g | Kohlenhydrate: 28g | Protein: 2g | Zucker: 20g | Natrium: 20mg

Kapitel 7: Snacks und Mahlzeiten für zwischendurch

Snacks zur Reduzierung von Entzündungen

80. Gurken-Hummus-Röllchen

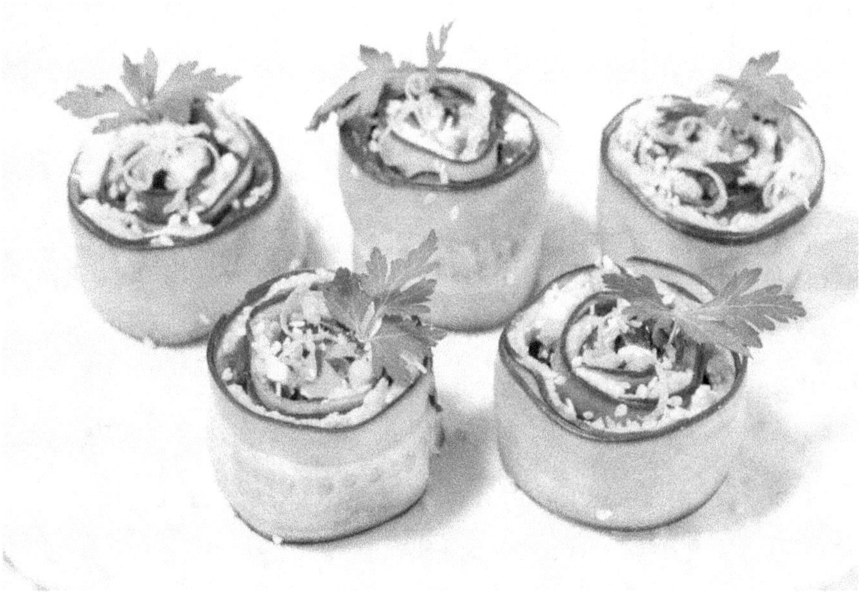

Zubereitungszeit: 15 Minuten | Kochzeit: 0 Minuten | Portionen: 2

Schwierigkeiten: Einfach

Zutaten:

- 1 große Gurke
- 4 EL Hummus
- 1 rote Paprika, in dünne Streifen geschnitten
- 1 Karotte, in dünne Streifen geschnitten
- 1 Handvoll frische Kresse
- Salz und Pfeffer nach Geschmack

Zubereitung:

1. Die Gurke der Länge nach in dünne Scheiben schneiden.
2. Jede Gurkenscheibe mit Hummus bestreichen.
3. Paprika- und Karottenstreifen sowie Kresse auf die Gurkenscheiben legen.

4. Die Gurkenscheiben vorsichtig aufrollen und mit einem Zahnstocher fixieren.
5. Mit Salz und Pfeffer abschmecken und sofort servieren.

Nährwerte (pro Portion): Kalorien: 120 | Fett: 6g | Kohlenhydrate: 12g | Protein: 3g | Zucker: 4g | Natrium: 220mg

81. Avocado-Ei-Salat auf Vollkornbrot

Zubereitungszeit: 10 Minuten | Kochzeit: 10 Minuten | Portionen: 2

Schwierigkeiten: Einfach

Zutaten:

- 2 Scheiben Vollkornbrot
- 1 reife Avocado
- 2 gekochte Eier
- 1 TL Zitronensaft
- Salz und Pfeffer nach Geschmack
- Eine Handvoll Rucola

Zubereitung:

1. Die Avocado schälen, entkernen und das Fruchtfleisch in einer Schüssel zerdrücken.
2. Die gekochten Eier schälen und in kleine Stücke schneiden.
3. Die Avocado mit den Eiern vermischen und Zitronensaft, Salz und Pfeffer hinzufügen.
4. Die Mischung auf die Vollkornbrotscheiben verteilen.
5. Mit Rucola garnieren und servieren.

Nährwerte (pro Portion): Kalorien: 250 | Fett: 15g | Kohlenhydrate: 22g | Protein: 8g | Zucker: 2g | Natrium: 300mg

82. Blaubeer-Mandel-Energiebällchen

Zubereitungszeit: 15 Minuten | Kochzeit: 0 Minuten | Portionen: 2

Schwierigkeiten: Einfach

Zutaten:

- 100 g Mandeln
- 50 g getrocknete Blaubeeren
- 2 EL Kokosöl, geschmolzen
- 1 EL Ahornsirup
- 1 TL Vanilleextrakt

Zubereitung:

1. Die Mandeln und getrockneten Blaubeeren in einem Mixer fein zerkleinern.
2. Kokosöl, Ahornsirup und Vanilleextrakt hinzufügen und zu einer klebrigen Masse vermischen.
3. Aus der Masse kleine Kugeln formen.
4. Die Energiebällchen im Kühlschrank fest werden lassen.
5. Nach Bedarf genießen.

Nährwerte (pro Portion): Kalorien: 220 | Fett: 15g | Kohlenhydrate: 18g | Protein: 5g | Zucker: 10g | Natrium: 10mg

83. Quinoa-Salat mit Granatapfel und Walnüssen

Zubereitungszeit: 15 Minuten | Kochzeit: 15 Minuten | Portionen: 2

Schwierigkeiten: Mittel

Zutaten:

- 100 g Quinoa
- 200 ml Wasser
- 1 Granatapfel, entkernt
- 50 g Walnüsse, gehackt
- 1 Handvoll Petersilie, gehackt
- 2 EL Zitronensaft
- 1 EL Olivenöl (nicht erhitzt)
- Salz und Pfeffer nach Geschmack

Zubereitung:

1. Die Quinoa in einem Sieb abspülen und mit Wasser in einem Topf zum Kochen bringen. 15 Minuten köcheln lassen, bis die Quinoa weich ist und das Wasser absorbiert wurde. Abkühlen lassen.
2. Die abgekühlte Quinoa in eine große Schüssel geben und mit Granatapfelkernen, Walnüssen und gehackter Petersilie vermischen.
3. Zitronensaft und Olivenöl hinzufügen und gut vermischen.
4. Mit Salz und Pfeffer abschmecken.
5. Sofort servieren oder im Kühlschrank aufbewahren.

Nährwerte (pro Portion): Kalorien: 250 | Fett: 14g | Kohlenhydrate: 28g | Protein: 6g | Zucker: 10g | Natrium: 40mg

84. Edamame mit Meersalz und Limette

Zubereitungszeit: 5 Minuten | Kochzeit: 5 Minuten | Portionen: 2

Schwierigkeiten: Einfach

Zutaten:

- 200 g Edamame (grüne Sojabohnen in der Schote)
- 1 TL Meersalz
- Saft von 1 Limette

Zubereitung:

1. Die Edamame in einem Topf mit kochendem Wasser 5 Minuten garen, bis sie weich sind.
2. Abgießen und in eine Schüssel geben.
3. Mit Meersalz und Limettensaft bestreuen und gut vermischen.
4. Sofort servieren.

Nährwerte (pro Portion): Kalorien: 120 | Fett: 4g | Kohlenhydrate: 10g | Protein: 10g | Zucker: 2g | Natrium: 300mg

85. Karottensticks mit Tahini-Dip

Zubereitungszeit: 10 Minuten | Kochzeit: 0 Minuten | Portionen: 2

Schwierigkeiten: Einfach

Zutaten:

- 4 Karotten, in Sticks geschnitten
- 2 EL Tahini
- 1 EL Zitronensaft
- 1 TL Ahornsirup
- 1 Knoblauchzehe, gehackt
- Salz und Pfeffer nach Geschmack

Zubereitung:

1. Die Karotten in Sticks schneiden und auf einen Teller legen.
2. In einer kleinen Schüssel Tahini, Zitronensaft, Ahornsirup, gehackten Knoblauch, Salz und Pfeffer zu einer glatten Sauce verrühren.
3. Den Tahini-Dip in ein Schälchen geben und mit den Karottensticks servieren.
4. Sofort genießen.

Nährwerte (pro Portion): Kalorien: 180 | Fett: 10g | Kohlenhydrate: 20g | Protein: 4g | Zucker: 8g | Natrium: 60mg

86. Apfelscheiben mit Mandelmus

Zubereitungszeit: 5 Minuten | Kochzeit: 0 Minuten | Portionen: 2

Schwierigkeiten: Einfach

Zutaten:

- 2 Äpfel
- 4 EL Mandelmus (ohne Zuckerzusatz)
- 1 TL Zimt

Zubereitung:

1. Die Äpfel in dünne Scheiben schneiden und auf einem Teller anrichten.
2. Das Mandelmus in einer kleinen Schüssel mit Zimt vermischen.
3. Das Mandelmus über die Apfelscheiben träufeln.
4. Sofort servieren.

Nährwerte (pro Portion): Kalorien: 220 | Fett: 12g | Kohlenhydrate: 24g | Protein: 4g | Zucker: 18g | Natrium: 0mg

87. Grünkohlchips

Zubereitungszeit: 10 Minuten | Kochzeit: 15 Minuten | Portionen: 2

Schwierigkeiten: Einfach

Zutaten:

- 1 Bund Grünkohl
- 1 EL Olivenöl (nicht erhitzt)
- 1 TL Meersalz
- 1 TL Paprikapulver

Zubereitung:

1. Den Ofen auf 180 Grad vorheizen.
2. Den Grünkohl waschen, trocken tupfen und in mundgerechte Stücke reißen.
3. In einer Schüssel Grünkohl mit Olivenöl, Meersalz und Paprikapulver vermischen.
4. Die Grünkohlstücke auf einem Backblech verteilen und 15 Minuten backen, bis sie knusprig sind.
5. Sofort servieren.

Nährwerte (pro Portion): Kalorien: 90 | Fett: 5g | Kohlenhydrate: 8g | Protein: 3g | Zucker: 1g | Natrium: 200mg

88. Beeren-Joghurt-Parfait

Zubereitungszeit: 10 Minuten | Kochzeit: 0 Minuten | Portionen: 2

Schwierigkeiten: Einfach

Zutaten:

- 200 g griechischer Joghurt
- 100 g gemischte Beeren (frisch oder gefroren)
- 2 EL gehackte Mandeln
- 1 TL Honig

Zubereitung:

1. Den griechischen Joghurt in zwei Gläser füllen.
2. Die Beeren gleichmäßig auf den Joghurt verteilen.

3. Mit gehackten Mandeln bestreuen.
4. Einen Teelöffel Honig über jedes Glas träufeln.
5. Sofort servieren.

Nährwerte (pro Portion): Kalorien: 180 | Fett: 8g | Kohlenhydrate: 20g | Protein: 10g | Zucker: 15g | Natrium: 40mg

89. Avocado-Kakaopudding

Zubereitungszeit: 10 Minuten | Kochzeit: 0 Minuten | Portionen: 2

Schwierigkeiten: Einfach

Zutaten:

- 2 reife Avocados
- 3 EL ungesüßtes Kakaopulver
- 2 EL Ahornsirup
- 1 TL Vanilleextrakt
- Eine Prise Salz

Zubereitung:

1. Die Avocados schälen und entkernen.
2. Das Avocado-Fruchtfleisch zusammen mit Kakaopulver, Ahornsirup, Vanilleextrakt und Salz in einen Mixer geben.
3. Zu einer glatten Masse pürieren.
4. Den Pudding in Dessertschalen füllen und mindestens 30 Minuten im Kühlschrank kühlen.
5. Sofort servieren.

Nährwerte (pro Portion): Kalorien: 250 | Fett: 18g | Kohlenhydrate: 25g | Protein: 3g | Zucker: 10g | Natrium: 50mg

Schnelle und einfache Optionen

90. Paprika- und Hummus-Sticks

Zubereitungszeit: 10 Minuten | Kochzeit: 0 Minuten | Portionen: 2

Schwierigkeiten: Einfach

Zutaten:

- 2 rote Paprika
- 4 EL Hummus
- 1 TL Olivenöl (nicht erhitzt)
- 1 TL Zitronensaft
- Salz und Pfeffer nach Geschmack

Zubereitung:

1. Die Paprika in Streifen schneiden.
2. Den Hummus in eine kleine Schüssel geben und mit Olivenöl und Zitronensaft verrühren.
3. Mit Salz und Pfeffer abschmecken.
4. Die Paprikastreifen mit dem Hummus-Dip servieren.

Nährwerte (pro Portion): Kalorien: 150 | Fett: 8g | Kohlenhydrate: 15g | Protein: 4g | Zucker: 6g | Natrium: 180mg

91. Apfel-Zimt-Reisflocken

Zubereitungszeit: 5 Minuten | Kochzeit: 0 Minuten | Portionen: 2

Schwierigkeiten: Einfach

Zutaten:

- 2 Äpfel, in dünne Scheiben geschnitten
- 4 EL Reisflocken
- 1 TL Zimt
- 1 TL Ahornsirup
- 1 TL Zitronensaft

Zubereitung:

1. Die Apfelscheiben auf einem Teller anrichten.
2. Reisflocken über die Apfelscheiben streuen.

3. Zimt und Zitronensaft darüber geben.
4. Mit Ahornsirup beträufeln und servieren.

Nährwerte (pro Portion): Kalorien: 140 | Fett: 1g | Kohlenhydrate: 33g | Protein: 1g | Zucker: 22g | Natrium: 5mg

92. Nussige Snack-Mischung

Zubereitungszeit: 5 Minuten | Kochzeit: 0 Minuten | Portionen: 2

Schwierigkeiten: Einfach

Zutaten:

- 50 g Mandeln
- 50 g Walnüsse
- 50 g getrocknete Cranberries
- 2 EL Kürbiskerne
- 1 TL Zimt

Zubereitung:

1. Alle Zutaten in eine Schüssel geben.
2. Gut vermischen.
3. In kleine Schälchen füllen und genießen.

Nährwerte (pro Portion): Kalorien: 300 | Fett: 24g | Kohlenhydrate: 16g | Protein: 8g | Zucker: 10g | Natrium: 5mg

93. Beeren-Kokos-Smoothie

Zubereitungszeit: 5 Minuten | Kochzeit: 0 Minuten | Portionen: 2

Schwierigkeiten: Einfach

Zutaten:

- 200 g gemischte Beeren (frisch oder gefroren)
- 200 ml Kokosmilch
- 1 Banane
- 1 TL Ahornsirup
- 1 TL Chiasamen

Zubereitung:

1. Die Beeren, Kokosmilch, Banane und Ahornsirup in einen Mixer geben.

2. Zu einem glatten Smoothie pürieren.
3. In Gläser füllen und mit Chiasamen bestreuen.
4. Sofort servieren.

Nährwerte (pro Portion): Kalorien: 180 | Fett: 8g | Kohlenhydrate: 28g | Protein: 2g | Zucker: 18g | Natrium: 10mg

94. Avocado-Tomaten-Toast

Zubereitungszeit: 10 Minuten | Kochzeit: 5 Minuten | Portionen: 2

Schwierigkeiten: Einfach

Zutaten:

- 2 Scheiben Vollkornbrot
- 1 reife Avocado
- 1 Tomate, in Scheiben geschnitten
- 1 TL Zitronensaft
- Salz und Pfeffer nach Geschmack

Zubereitung:

1. Das Vollkornbrot im Toaster leicht anrösten.
2. Die Avocado schälen, entkernen und das Fruchtfleisch in einer Schüssel zerdrücken.
3. Zitronensaft, Salz und Pfeffer zur Avocado hinzufügen und gut vermischen.
4. Die Avocadomischung auf die gerösteten Brotscheiben streichen.
5. Mit Tomatenscheiben belegen und servieren.

Nährwerte (pro Portion): Kalorien: 220 | Fett: 14g | Kohlenhydrate: 20g | Protein: 4g | Zucker: 2g | Natrium: 150mg

95. Mango-Kokos-Energieballs

Zubereitungszeit: 15 Minuten | Kochzeit: 0 Minuten | Portionen: 2

Schwierigkeiten: Einfach

Zutaten:

- 100 g getrocknete Mangostücke
- 50 g Mandeln
- 2 EL Kokosflocken
- 1 TL Vanilleextrakt

Zubereitung:

1. Die getrockneten Mangostücke und Mandeln in einem Mixer fein zerkleinern.
2. Kokosflocken und Vanilleextrakt hinzufügen und gut vermischen.
3. Aus der Masse kleine Kugeln formen.
4. Im Kühlschrank fest werden lassen und nach Bedarf genießen.

Nährwerte (pro Portion): Kalorien: 250 | Fett: 12g | Kohlenhydrate: 30g | Protein: 4g | Zucker: 20g | Natrium: 5mg

96. Kürbiskern- und Cranberry-Riegel

Zubereitungszeit: 10 Minuten | Kochzeit: 10 Minuten | Portionen: 2

Schwierigkeiten: Mittel

Zutaten:

- 100 g Haferflocken
- 50 g Kürbiskerne
- 50 g getrocknete Cranberries
- 2 EL Ahornsirup
- 1 TL Zimt

Zubereitung:

1. Den Ofen auf 180 Grad vorheizen.
2. Haferflocken, Kürbiskerne, getrocknete Cranberries, Ahornsirup und Zimt in einer Schüssel gut vermischen.
3. Die Mischung auf ein Backblech drücken und gleichmäßig verteilen.
4. 10 Minuten backen, bis die Riegel goldbraun sind.
5. Abkühlen lassen, in Riegel schneiden und servieren.

Nährwerte (pro Portion): Kalorien: 220 | Fett: 10g | Kohlenhydrate: 30g | Protein: 6g | Zucker: 12g | Natrium: 5mg

97. Erdnussbutter-Äpfel

Zubereitungszeit: 5 Minuten | Kochzeit: 0 Minuten | Portionen: 2

Schwierigkeiten: Einfach

Zutaten:

- 2 Äpfel
- 4 EL Erdnussbutter (ohne Zuckerzusatz)
- 1 TL Zimt

Zubereitung:

1. Die Äpfel in dünne Scheiben schneiden.
2. Die Erdnussbutter in einer kleinen Schüssel mit Zimt vermischen.
3. Die Apfelscheiben mit der Zimt-Erdnussbutter bestreichen.
4. Sofort servieren.

Nährwerte (pro Portion): Kalorien: 200 | Fett: 12g | Kohlenhydrate: 22g | Protein: 4g | Zucker: 16g | Natrium: 0mg

98. Wassermelonen-Feta-Salat

Zubereitungszeit: 10 Minuten | Kochzeit: 0 Minuten | Portionen: 2

Schwierigkeiten: Einfach

Zutaten:

- 200 g Wassermelone, gewürfelt
- 50 g Feta-Käse, zerbröckelt
- 1 EL frische Minze, gehackt
- 1 EL Zitronensaft
- 1 TL Olivenöl (nicht erhitzt)
- Salz und Pfeffer nach Geschmack

Zubereitung:

1. Die gewürfelte Wassermelone und den zerbröckelten Feta in eine Schüssel geben.
2. Die gehackte Minze, Zitronensaft und Olivenöl hinzufügen.
3. Mit Salz und Pfeffer abschmecken.
4. Gut vermischen und sofort servieren.

Nährwerte (pro Portion): Kalorien: 140 | Fett: 8g | Kohlenhydrate: 14g | Protein: 4g | Zucker: 10g | Natrium: 180mg

99. Zucchini-Chips

Zubereitungszeit: 10 Minuten | Kochzeit: 30 Minuten | Portionen: 2

Schwierigkeiten: Einfach

Zutaten:

- 2 Zucchini, in dünne Scheiben geschnitten
- 1 EL Olivenöl (nicht erhitzt)
- 1 TL Meersalz
- 1 TL Paprikapulver

Zubereitung:

1. Den Ofen auf 150 Grad vorheizen.
2. Die Zucchinischeiben in eine Schüssel geben und mit Olivenöl, Meersalz und Paprikapulver vermischen.
3. Die Zucchinischeiben auf einem Backblech ausbreiten.
4. 30 Minuten backen, bis die Zucchini knusprig sind.
5. Sofort servieren.

Nährwerte (pro Portion): Kalorien: 90 | Fett: 5g | Kohlenhydrate: 10g | Protein: 2g | Zucker: 2g | Natrium: 220mg

100. Kichererbsen-Avocado-Salat

Zubereitungszeit: 10 Minuten | Kochzeit: 0 Minuten | Portionen: 2

Schwierigkeiten: Einfach

Zutaten:

- 1 Dose Kichererbsen (400 g), abgetropft und gespült
- 1 reife Avocado, gewürfelt
- 1 kleine rote Zwiebel, fein gehackt
- 1 Handvoll Kirschtomaten, halbiert
- 1 EL Zitronensaft
- 1 EL Olivenöl (nicht erhitzt)
- Salz und Pfeffer nach Geschmack
- 1 Handvoll frische Petersilie, gehackt

Zubereitung:

1. Die abgetropften Kichererbsen in eine Schüssel geben.

2. Die gewürfelte Avocado, gehackte Zwiebel und halbierten Kirschtomaten hinzufügen.
3. Zitronensaft und Olivenöl über den Salat geben und gut vermischen.
4. Mit Salz und Pfeffer abschmecken.
5. Mit gehackter Petersilie bestreuen und sofort servieren.

Nährwerte (pro Portion): Kalorien: 280 | Fett: 16g | Kohlenhydrate: 28g | Protein: 6g | Zucker: 4g | Natrium: 220mg

Kapitel 8: 30-Tage-Essensplan und Einkaufsliste

30-Tage-Essensplan

Tag	Frühstück	Mittagessen	Abendessen	Snack
1	Heidelbeer-Chia-Pudding	Quinoa-Gemüse-Bowl	Gebackener Lachs mit Gemüse	Gurken-Hummus-Röllchen
2	Avocado-Toast mit Tomaten und Kresse	Linsensalat mit Rote Bete und Walnüssen	Quinoa-Bowl mit gebratenem Gemüse und Tahini-Sauce	Avocado-Ei-Salat auf Vollkornbrot
3	Grüner Smoothie mit Spinat und Ananas	Kichererbsen-Curry mit Spinat	Gefüllte Champignons mit Spinat und Kichererbsen	Blaubeer-Mandel-Energiebällchen
4	Haferflocken mit Apfel und Zimt	Gebackene Süßkartoffel mit Avocado-Salsa	Ofen-Gemüse mit Rosmarin	Quinoa-Salat mit Granatapfel und Walnüssen
5	Quinoa-Frühstücksschale mit Beeren	Mediterrane Kichererbsen-Bowl	Tomaten-Basilikum-Suppe	Edamame mit Meersalz und Limette
6	Mandel- und Blaubeer-Muffins	Blumenkohl-Reis mit Erbsen und Minze	Gebackene Aubergine mit Knoblauch-Joghurt-Sauce	Karottensticks mit Tahini-Dip
7	Buchweizen-Pfannkuchen mit Beerenkompott	Tofu-Gemüse-Pfanne	Kichererbsen-Curry mit Kokosmilch	Apfelscheiben mit Mandelmus
8	Kokosnuss-Granola mit Joghurt	Quinoa-Tabouleh mit Granatapfel	Spaghetti aus Zucchini mit Tomaten und	Grünkohlchips

			Basilikum	
9	Bircher Müsli	Vegane Linsensuppe	Linseneintopf mit Gemüse	Beeren-Joghurt-Parfait
10	Süßkartoffel-Toast mit Avocado und Ei	Gebackene Aubergine mit Tomaten und Tahini	Gebratene Pilze mit Kräutern	Avocado-Kakaopudding
11	Matcha-Grüner-Smoothie-Bowl	Sommerlicher Gemüsesalat mit Zitronen-Dressing	Linsensalat mit geröstetem Gemüse	Paprika- und Hummus-Sticks
12	Quinoa-Obstsalat	Zucchini-Nudeln mit Pesto	Blumenkohl-Curry mit Kokosmilch	Apfel-Zimt-Reisflocken
13	Süßkartoffel- und Avocado-Brei	Gebackene Paprika mit Quinoa-Füllung	Zucchini-Lasagne mit Spinat	Nussige Snack-Mischung
14	Hirsebrei mit Beeren	Blumenkohl-Steak mit Tahini-Dressing	Kichererbsen-Bowl mit gebratenem Gemüse	Beeren-Kokos-Smoothie
15	Mandel- und Kokos-Joghurtparfait	Gurken-Avocado-Suppe	Gebratener Tofu mit Sesam und Brokkoli	Avocado-Tomaten-Toast
16	Zucchini- und Möhrenpuffer	Rote-Bete-Carpaccio mit Walnüssen	Quinoa-Salat mit Avocado und Mango	Mango-Kokos-Energieballs
17	Chia-Pudding mit Mango und Kokos	Gebackener Tofu mit Sesam und Frühlingszwiebeln	Gebackene Süßkartoffeln mit Tahini-Dressing	Kürbiskern- und Cranberry-Riegel
18	Buchweizen-Müsli mit Äpfeln und Nüssen	Spinat-Salat mit Granatapfel und Mandeln	Spinat-Curry mit Kichererbsen	Erdnussbutter-Äpfel
19	Hummus-Toast mit Paprika und	Linsensalat mit Mango und	Gebackene Aubergine mit	Wassermelonen-Feta-Salat

	Kresse	Avocado	Tomaten und Basilikum	
20	Tofu-Rührei mit Spinat und Tomaten	Auberginen-Röllchen mit Spinat und Pinienkernen	Karotten-Ingwer-Suppe	Zucchini-Chips
21	Heidelbeer-Chia-Pudding	Quinoa-Gemüse-Bowl	Gebackener Lachs mit Gemüse	Gurken-Hummus-Röllchen
22	Avocado-Toast mit Tomaten und Kresse	Linsensalat mit Rote Bete und Walnüssen	Quinoa-Bowl mit gebratenem Gemüse und Tahini-Sauce	Avocado-Ei-Salat auf Vollkornbrot
23	Grüner Smoothie mit Spinat und Ananas	Kichererbsen-Curry mit Spinat	Gefüllte Champignons mit Spinat und Kichererbsen	Blaubeer-Mandel-Energiebällchen
24	Haferflocken mit Apfel und Zimt	Gebackene Süßkartoffel mit Avocado-Salsa	Ofen-Gemüse mit Rosmarin	Quinoa-Salat mit Granatapfel und Walnüssen
25	Quinoa-Frühstücksschale mit Beeren	Mediterrane Kichererbsen-Bowl	Tomaten-Basilikum-Suppe	Edamame mit Meersalz und Limette
26	Mandel- und Blaubeer-Muffins	Blumenkohl-Reis mit Erbsen und Minze	Gebackene Aubergine mit Knoblauch-Joghurt-Sauce	Karottensticks mit Tahini-Dip
27	Buchweizen-Pfannkuchen mit Beerenkompott	Tofu-Gemüse-Pfanne	Kichererbsen-Curry mit Kokosmilch	Apfelscheiben mit Mandelmus
28	Kokosnuss-Granola mit Joghurt	Quinoa-Tabouleh mit Granatapfel	Spaghetti aus Zucchini mit Tomaten und Basilikum	Grünkohlchips

29	Bircher Müsli	Vegane Linsensuppe	Linseneintopf mit Gemüse	Beeren-Joghurt-Parfait
30	Süßkartoffel-Toast mit Avocado und Ei	Gebackene Aubergine mit Tomaten und Tahini	Gebratene Pilze mit Kräutern	Avocado-Kakaopudding

Einkaufsliste

Obst und Gemüse

- Heidelbeeren (Blaubeeren) - 400 g
- Avocados - 20
- Tomaten - 20
- Kresse - 2 Handvoll
- Spinat - 1 kg
- Ananas - 4
- Äpfel - 10
- Zimt - 1 kleines Glas
- Beeren (gemischt) - 800 g
- Süßkartoffeln - 12
- Granatäpfel - 10
- Zitronen - 10
- Rote Bete - 6
- Blumenkohl - 6
- Gurken - 5
- Paprika - 10
- Karotten - 20
- Walnüsse - 300 g
- Limetten - 6
- Zucchini - 15
- Mangos - 8
- Kirschtomaten - 20
- Rote Zwiebeln - 20
- Zwiebeln - 20
- Ingwer - 200 g
- Knoblauchzehen - 15
- Erbsen - 200 g
- Minze - 3 Handvoll
- Auberginen - 6
- Petersilie - 6 Handvoll

- Kichererbsen (Dosen) - 20
- Koriander - 2 Handvoll
- Frühlingszwiebeln - 6
- Grünkohl - 4 Bund
- Mandeln - 500 g
- Hirse - 400 g
- Rucola - 3 Handvoll
- Granatapfelkerne - 6 Packungen
- Mandarinen - 4
- Bananen - 6
- Birnen - 6
- Erdnussbutter - 1 Glas
- Kirschen - 400 g

Getreide und Hülsenfrüchte

- Chiasamen - 200 g
- Quinoa - 1 kg
- Haferflocken - 500 g
- Buchweizenmehl - 500 g
- Reisflocken - 200 g
- Mandeln - 500 g
- Kokosflocken - 200 g
- Kürbiskerne - 200 g
- Hirse - 200 g
- Linsen (grün und rot) - 1 kg
- Kichererbsen (Dosen) - 10 Dosen

Milchprodukte und Ersatzprodukte

- Griechischer Joghurt - 2 kg
- Mandelmilch - 2 Liter
- Kokosmilch - 8 Dosen (400 ml)
- Tahini - 1 Glas
- Tofu - 2 kg

- Ricotta - 200 g
- Parmesan - 100 g
- Vanilleextrakt - 1 Flasche

Nüsse und Samen

- Walnüsse - 200 g
- Mandeln - 300 g
- Pinienkerne - 200 g
- Kürbiskerne - 200 g
- Sesamsamen - 200 g
- Kokosflocken - 200 g

Gewürze und Saucen

- Zimt - 1 Glas
- Kreuzkümmel - 1 Glas
- Paprika - 1 Glas
- Kurkuma - 1 Glas
- Pfeffer - 1 Glas
- Meersalz - 1 Glas
- Balsamico-Essig - 1 Flasche
- Olivenöl - 1 Liter (für kalte Gerichte)
- Ahornsirup - 1 Flasche
- Honig - 1 Glas
- Limettensaft - 1 Flasche
- Zitronensaft - 1 Flasche
- Sojasauce (natriumarm) - 1 Flasche
- Sesamöl - 1 Flasche

Fisch und Fleisch

- Lachsfilets - 1,5 kg

Sonstiges

- Kokosöl - 1 Glas

- Kakaopulver (ungesüßt) - 200 g
- Vanilleextrakt - 1 Flasche

Schlussfolgerungen

Abschließend lässt sich sagen, dass die Reise zu einer entzündungshemmenden Ernährungsweise nicht nur eine Veränderung in der Auswahl der Lebensmittel darstellt, sondern eine umfassende Lebensstilentscheidung ist, die zahlreiche Vorteile für die Gesundheit und das Wohlbefinden bietet. Diese Ernährung ist mehr als nur eine Diät; sie ist ein Weg, um den Körper mit den notwendigen Nährstoffen zu versorgen, die Entzündungen entgegenwirken und gleichzeitig Energie und Vitalität fördern.

Während der Entstehung dieses Buches haben wir verschiedene Aspekte dieser Ernährungsweise erkundet und praktische Ansätze vorgestellt, um sie in den Alltag zu integrieren

. Es ist ermutigend zu sehen, wie wissenschaftliche Erkenntnisse und kulinarische Kreativität Hand in Hand gehen, um eine gesunde und schmackhafte Ernährung zu fördern.

Ein wesentlicher Bestandteil dieser Ernährungsweise ist die Vielfalt der Lebensmittel, die in den täglichen Speiseplan integriert werden. Frisches Gemüse, Obst, Nüsse, Samen und gesunde Fette sind die Bausteine einer entzündungshemmenden Ernährung. Diese Lebensmittel bieten nicht nur eine Fülle von Nährstoffen, sondern auch verschiedene Aromen und Texturen, die das Essen zu einem genussvollen Erlebnis machen.

Die positiven Auswirkungen einer solchen Ernährung sind weitreichend. Viele Menschen berichten von einer spürbaren Verbesserung ihres allgemeinen Wohlbefindens, einschließlich erhöhter Energie, besserer Verdauung und weniger Entzündungssymptomen. Langfristig kann diese Ernährungsweise das Risiko für chronische Krankheiten wie Herz-Kreislauf-Erkrankungen, Diabetes und bestimmte Krebsarten erheblich reduzieren.

Die in diesem Buch vorgestellten Rezepte zeigen, wie vielfältig und lecker eine entzündungshemmende Ernährung sein kann. Von Frühstücksoptionen, die den Tag mit Energie starten lassen, über nährstoffreiche Mittag- und Abendessen bis hin zu süßen, aber gesunden Desserts und Snacks – jede Mahlzeit ist darauf ausgelegt, den Körper mit wichtigen Nährstoffen zu versorgen und gleichzeitig den Gaumen zu erfreuen.

Besonders wichtig ist, dass diese Ernährungsweise keine kurzfristige Diät ist, sondern eine langfristige Lebensstiländerung. Es geht darum, bewusste Entscheidungen zu treffen und Lebensmittel zu wählen, die den Körper nähren und stärken. Dies erfordert vielleicht einige Anpassungen und die Bereitschaft, neue Rezepte und Zubereitungsmethoden auszuprobieren.

Doch die positiven Auswirkungen auf die Gesundheit und das Wohlbefinden machen diese Anstrengungen lohnenswert.

Ein weiterer wichtiger Aspekt ist die Rolle, die diese Ernährungsweise in der Vorbeugung und Behandlung von Entzündungen spielt. Chronische Entzündungen sind oft ein stiller Auslöser für viele ernsthafte Gesundheitsprobleme. Durch die Wahl entzündungshemmender Lebensmittel können wir aktiv dazu beitragen, Entzündungen zu reduzieren und das Risiko für damit verbundene Krankheiten zu verringern.

Abschließend ist es wichtig zu betonen, dass jeder Einzelne die Macht hat, durch bewusste Ernährungsentscheidungen einen positiven Einfluss auf seine Gesundheit zu nehmen. Die in diesem Buch vorgestellten Rezepte und Tipps bieten eine solide Grundlage, um mit einer entzündungshemmenden Ernährung zu beginnen oder diese weiter zu vertiefen. Es erfordert Engagement und Achtsamkeit, aber die Vorteile sind enorm.

SCANNEN SIE DEN QR-CODE FÜR SOFORTIGEN ZUGANG ZU IHREM BONUS

www.ingramcontent.com/pod-product-compliance
Lightning Source LLC
Chambersburg PA
CBHW080435240526
45479CB00015B/1172
* 9 7 9 8 3 3 2 2 4 8 0 7 8 *

Note that the column fx is obtained by multiplying the values of numbers in the column f by numbers in the column x.

$$\text{Mean, } \bar{x} = \frac{\Sigma fx}{\Sigma f}$$

$$= \frac{155}{50}$$

$$= 3.1$$

(b) Since there are 50 students, i.e. the total frequency is 50, and 50 is an even number, then the positions of the two middle marks and their average are obtained as follows:

$$\text{Median} = \frac{Number\ \ in\ the\ \left(\frac{\Sigma f}{2}\right)th\ position\ + Number\ \ in\ the\ \left(\frac{\Sigma f + 2}{2}\right)th\ position}{2}$$

$$= \frac{Number\ \ in\ the\ \left(\frac{50}{2}\right)th\ position\ + Number\ \ in\ the\ \left(\frac{50+2}{2}\right)th\ position}{2}$$

$$= \frac{Number\ \ in\ the\ 25th\ position\ + Number\ \ in\ the\ \left(\frac{52}{2}\right)th\ position}{2}$$

$$= \frac{Number\ \ in\ the\ 25th\ position + Number\ \ in\ the\ 26th\ position}{2}$$

$= \frac{3+3}{2}$ (Note that 3 is the mark in the 25th position and in the 26th position)

$$= \frac{6}{2}$$

$$= 3$$

∴ The median is 3

Use the frequency (number of students) to locate the marks in the 25th and 26th position as follows: The first frequency of 8 shows that mark 1 occupies the position of 1st to 8th. Adding the second frequency of 16 to the first frequency gives, 8 + 16 = 24. This shows that after the 8th position occupied by the mark 1, the positions 9th to 24th is occupied by the mark 2. Adding the third frequency of 10 to the previous sum of frequencies gives, 10 + 24 = 34. This shows that after the 24th position occupied by the mark 2, the positions 25th to 34th is occupied by the mark 3. Hence, 3 is the mark in the 25th and 26th position which are at the middle of the data.

(c) The mode is the mark that has the highest frequency. From the table, the mark 2 has the highest frequency of 16. So, the mode is 2.

∴ The mode is 2.

Note that the mode is not the frequency itself, but that particular mark that has the highest frequency. Avoid the mistake of taking 16 (frequency) as the mode.

RANGE

Range is the difference between the highest and lowest values in a given set of data. It is a measure of dispersion or variation.

Example

Find the range of the following set of numbers: 4, 8, 2, 5, 8, 3, 6, 4, 9, 2, 5

Solution

The highest number in the data set is 9, while the lowest number is 2.

∴ Range = Highest number – Lowest number

$= 9 - 2 = 7$

Range = 7

Practice Questions

1. Find the mean, median and mode of the data below:
   1, 6, 10, 4, 1, 2, 5, 2, 3, 2, 8

Solution

2. Find: (a) the mean;

   (b) the median;

   (c) the mode of the data below.

   20, 24, 21, 25, 22, 25, 28, 26, 20, 23, 25, 27 and 26

Solution

3. Find the mean, median and mode of the data below:

101, 105, 120, 116, 109, 112, 118, 115, 105 and 111

Solution

4. Find the mean, median and mode of the data below:

   0, 6, 8, 2, 5, 9, 1, 5, 4, 7, 5, 2, 3, 3

Solution

5. The table below shows the marks of 50 students in a test.

Mark	3	4	5	6	7	8	9
No of Student	8	16	10	5	3	6	2

Calculate: (a) the mean (b) the median (c) the mode of the marks

Solution

6. The table below shows the ages of 30 students in a school.

Age	10	11	12	13	14	15
No of Student	1	4	3	7	9	6

Calculate: (a) the mean (b) the median (c) the mode of the ages

Solution

7. Find the range of the following set of data

(a) 12, 17, 21, 15, 19, 13, 11, 16, 22, 12, 13

(b) 231kg, 258kg, 213kg, 243kg, 216kg, 271kg, 262kg, 219kg, 238kg, 231kg.

Solution

(a)

(b)

Answers to Chapter 2

1. Mean = 4 Median = 3 Mode = 2

2. (a) 24 (b) 25 (c) 25

3. Mean = 111.2 Median = 111.5 Mode = 105

4. Mean = 4.3 Median = 4.5 Mode = 5

5. (a) 5.1 (b) 5 (c) 4

6. (a) 13.2 (b) 13.5 (c) 14

7. (a) 11 (b) 58kg

CHAPTER 3
COLLECTION AND TABULATION OF GROUPED DATA

Statistical data containing numerous values is easier to work with when the values are grouped into class intervals.

Example

The data below gives the marks of 30 students in an exam.

43	45	50	47	51	58	52	47	42	54
61	50	45	55	57	41	46	49	51	50
59	44	53	57	49	40	48	52	51	58

Taking class intervals 40 – 44, 45 – 49, ……, construct a frequency distribution for the data.

Solution

The data is summarized as shown on the table below. Note that the highest value in the given data falls within the range 60 – 64.

Class interval	40 - 44	45 - 49	50 - 54	55 - 59	60 - 64
Frequency	5	8	10	6	1

TERMS USED IN GROUPED DATA

The table below will be used to explain the terms used in grouped data.

Class interval	Frequency
8 – 14	3
15 – 21	5
22 – 28	8
29 – 35	18

1. Class limit: The end numbers in each class interval are called the class limits. 8 is the lower class limit, while 14 is the upper class limit of the first class interval.

2. Class boundaries: The class boundary for the second class interval is 14.5 – 21.5. The lower class boundary is 14.5 which is obtained by subtracting 0.5 from 15 (the lower class limit). The upper class

boundary is 21.5 which is obtained by adding 0.5 to 21 (the upper class limit). Other class boundaries are obtained in a similar way.

3. Class width: For each class interval the difference between the upper class boundary and the lower class boundary gives the class width. From the table above the class width for the third class interval is 28.5 – 21.5 = 7

4. Class mid-value: This is half of the sum of the lower and upper class limit of a given class interval. The class-value of the first class interval is given by: $\frac{8+14}{2} = \frac{22}{2} = 11.$

Example

Copy and complete the table below.

Class interval	Frequency	Class boundary	Class width	Class mid-value
55 – 59	3			
60 – 64	2			
65 – 69	5			
70 – 74	4			
75 – 79	1			

Solution

The completed table is as shown below

Class interval	Frequency	Class boundary	Class width	Class mid-value
55 – 59	3	54.5 – 59.5	5	57
60 – 64	2	59.5 – 64.5	5	62
65 – 69	5	64.5 – 69.5	5	67
70 – 74	4	69.5 – 74.5	5	72
75 – 79	1	74.5 – 79.5	5	77

Note that the class boundaries are obtained by subtracting and adding 0.5 to the lower and upper class limits respectively. This 0.5 is obtained by finding the difference between the lower class limit of one class and the upper class limit of the previous class and dividing the result by 2. This gives, for example (60 – 59)/2 = ½ = 0.5. The class width is the difference between the upper and lower class boundaries. The class mid-values are obtained by taking the mean of the upper and lower class limits.

Practice Questions

1. The data below gives the scores of 50 students in an exam.

43	45	50	47	51	58	52	47	42	54
61	50	45	55	57	41	46	49	51	50
59	44	53	57	49	40	48	52	51	58
48	54	43	54	61	60	49	57	45	42
56	45	57	61	54	62	44	47	46	62

Taking class intervals 40 – 44, 45 – 49, ..., construct a frequency distribution for the data.

Solution

2. The data below shows the weights in kg of students in a school.

24	32	44	51	31	23	51	34	48	40
53	45	29	35	27	51	29	35	50	30
43	55	53	35	26	28	41	44	54	43
27	45	33	41	55	28	32	51	26	39

Taking class intervals 21 – 25, 26 – 30, ..., construct a frequency table for the data.

Solution

3. Copy and complete the table below.

Class interval	Frequency	Class boundary	Class width	Class mid-value
5 – 9	2			
10 – 14	5			
15 – 19	5			
20 – 24	7			
25 – 29	1			

Solution

4. Copy and complete the table below.

Class interval	Frequency	Class boundary	Class width	Class mid-value
1 – 20	1			
21 – 40	4			

41 – 60	7			
61 – 80	3			
81 – 100	5			

Solution

5. Copy and complete the table below.

Class interval	Frequency	Class boundary	Class width	Class mid-value
0 – 90	2			
100 – 190	4			
200 – 290	1			
300 – 390	7			
400 – 490	1			

Solution

Answers to Chapter 3

1.

Score	40 - 44	45 - 49	50 - 54	55 - 59	60 – 64
Frequency	8	14	13	9	6

2.

Weight	21 - 25	26 - 30	31 - 35	36 - 40	41 - 45	46 - 50	51 – 55
Frequency	2	9	8	2	8	2	9

3.

Class interval	Frequency	Class Boundary	Class width	Class mid-value
5 – 9	2	4.5 – 9.5	20	7
10 – 14	5	9.5 – 14.5	20	12
15 – 19	5	14.5 – 19.5	20	17
20 – 24	7	19.5 – 24.5	20	22
25 – 29	1	24.5 – 29.5	20	27

4.

Class interval	Frequency	Class Boundary	Class width	Class mid-value
1 – 20	1	0.5 – 20.5	20	10.5
21 – 40	4	20.5 – 40.5	20	30.5
41 – 60	7	40.5 – 60.5	20	50.5
61 – 80	3	60.5 – 80.5	20	70.5
81 – 100	5	80.5 – 100.5	20	90.5

5.

Class interval	Frequency	Class Boundary	Class width	Class mid-value
0 – 90	2	-5 – 95	100	45
100 – 190	4	95 – 195	100	145

200 – 290	1	195 – 295	100	245
300 – 390	7	295 – 395	100	345
400 – 490	1	395 - 495	100	445

CHAPTER 4
MEAN, MEDIAN AND MODE OF GROUPED DATA

MEAN

The mean of a grouped data can be calculated by substituting thre class mid value as the values of x in the formula given by:

$$\text{Mean } \overline{X} = \frac{\sum fx}{\sum f}$$

MEDIAN

The median of a grouped data can be estimated by:

$$\text{Median} = L + C\left(\frac{\frac{\sum f}{2} - CF_{bm}}{F_m}\right)$$

Where, $\frac{\sum f}{2}$ determines the median class

L = Lower class boundary of the median class

CF_{bm} = Cumulative frequency before the median class

F_m = Frequency of the median class

C = Class width

MODE

The mode of a grouped data can be calculated as follows:

$$\text{Mode} = L + C\left(\frac{\Delta_1}{\Delta_1 + \Delta_2}\right)$$

Where, L = Lower class boundary of modal class

C = Class width

Δ_1 = Difference between the frequency of the modal class and the frequency before it

Δ_2 = Difference between the frequency of the modal class and the frequency after it

Example

The following table shows the frequency distribution of ages, in years of 50 people at a bus stop.

Ages	10 - 19	20 - 29	30 - 39	40 - 49	50 - 59	60 - 69
Number of people	6	12	16	9	5	2

Calculate: (a) the mean

(b) the median

(c) the mode of the distribution

Solution

Ages	Number of people (f)	Cumulative frequency	Class mid-value(x)	fx	Class boundary	Class width
10 – 19	6	6	14.5	87	9.5-19.5	10
20 – 29	12	6+12=18	24.5	294	19.5-29.5	10
30 – 39	16	18+16=34	34.5	552	29.5-39.5	10
40 – 49	9	34+9=43	44.5	400.5	39.5-49.5	10
50 – 59	5	43+5=48	54.5	272.5	49.5-59.5	10
60 – 69	2	48+2=50	64.5	129	59.5-69.5	10
	$\sum f = 50$			$\sum f = 1735$		

(a) Mean $\bar{X} = \frac{\sum fx}{\sum f}$

$= \frac{1735}{50} = 34.7$

(b) Median $= L + C(\frac{\frac{\sum f}{2} - CF_{bm}}{F_m})$

$\frac{\sum f}{2} = \frac{50}{2} = 25$

This shows that the median class falls in the 25th position

∴ Median class = 30 – 39

Lower class boundary of median class, L = 29.5

Class width, C = 10

Cumulative frequency before the median class, $CF_{bm} = 18$

Frequency of the median class, $F_m = 16$

∴ Median $= L + C(\frac{\frac{\sum f}{2} - CF_{bm}}{F_m})$

$= 29.5 + 10(\frac{25 - 18}{16})$

$= 29.5 + 10(\frac{7}{16})$

$= 29.5 + 4.375 = 33.875$

$\therefore$ Median = 33.9 (To 1 d.p)

(c) Mode = $L + C(\frac{\Delta_1}{\Delta_1 + \Delta_2})$

Modal class = 30 – 39

Lower class boundary of modal class, L = 29.5

Class width = 10

Δ_1 = Modal class frequency – frequency before it

= 16 - 12 = 4

Δ_2 = Modal class frequency – frequency after it

= 16 - 9 = 7

$\therefore$ Mode = $L + C(\frac{\Delta_1}{\Delta_1 + \Delta_2})$

$= 29.5 + 10(\frac{4}{4+7})$

$= 29.5 + 10(\frac{4}{11})$

$= 29.5 + 3.64 = 33.14$

$\therefore$ Mode = 33.1 (To 1 d.p)

Practice Questions

1. The following table shows the weights of 30 people at a company.

Weight	60 - 64	65 - 69	70 - 74	75 - 79	80 - 84	85 - 89
Number of people	1	12	7	5	3	2

Calculate: (a) the mean

(b) the median

(c) the mode of the distribution

2. The data below is the load distribution in tones, a chain can support.

Load	83 - 85	86 - 88	89 - 91	92 - 94	95 - 97
Number of chain	2	8	5	14	1

Determine: (a) the mean

(b) the median

(c) the mode of the weights

Solution

(a)

(b)

(c)

2. The data below is the ages, in years, of 50 people at a party.

Ages	1 - 20	21 - 40	41 - 60	61 - 80	81-100
Number of people	3	21	17	7	2

Determine: (a) the mean

(b) the median

(c) the mode of the weights

Solution

(a)

(b)

(c)

Answers to Chapter 4

1. (a) 72.5	(b) 70.9	(c) 67.9
2. (a) 90.4	(b) 91.5	(c) 92.7
3. (a) 44.1	(b) 41.7	(c) 36.9

CHAPTER 5
MEAN DEVIATION

The mean deviation of a set of data is the mean of the absolute deviation of the values from the mean of the group. The mean deviation for data not given in a frequency table is given by:

Mean deviation = $\frac{\sum |x - \bar{x}|}{N}$ where x is each value in the data, $\bar{X}$, is the mean and N is the number of values in the data.

For data given in a frequency table, the mean deviation is given by:

Mean deviation = $\frac{\sum f|x - \bar{x}|}{\sum f}$

Examples

1. Calculate the mean deviation of the following data: 2, 4, 1, 3, 0

Solution

Let us first calculate the mean of the data.

Mean, $\bar{x} = \frac{2 + 4 + 1 + 3 + 0}{5} = \frac{10}{5} = 2$

$\therefore\ \bar{x} = 2$

The deviation from the mean ($x - \bar{x}$) is now tabulated as follows.

Data (x)	$x - \bar{x}$ ($\bar{x} = 2$)	$\lvert x - \bar{x} \rvert$
2	0	0
4	2	2
1	-1	1
3	1	1
0	-2	2
		$\sum \lvert x - \bar{x} \rvert = 6$

$\therefore$ Mean deviation = $\frac{\sum |x - \bar{x}|}{N} = \frac{6}{5} = 1.2$

2. The marks obtained by 40 students in a mathematics test are as shown below. Calculate the mean deviation of the data.

Marks	31 - 40	41 - 50	51 – 60	61 - 70	71 - 80	81 - 90	91- 100
Number of student	1	2	8	11	8	6	4

Solution

The table below summarizes the determination of the mean and the values needed for the mean deviation. Note that the mean used on the table has been calculated below the table.

Mark	mid-value x	$x - \bar{x}$ $\bar{x} = 69.75$	$\lvert x - \bar{x}\rvert$	No of student f	fx	$f\lvert x - \bar{x}\rvert$
31 – 40	35.5	-34.25	34.25	1	35.5	34.25
41 – 50	45.5	-24.25	24.25	2	91	48.50
51 – 60	55.5	-14.24	14.24	8	444	114
61 – 70	65.5	-4.25	4.25	11	720.5	46.75
71 – 80	75.5	5.75	5.75	8	604	46
81 – 90	85.5	15.75	15.75	6	513	94.5
91 – 100	95.5	25.75	25.75	4	382	103
				$\sum f = 40$	$\sum fx = 2790$	

Mean, $\bar{x} = \frac{\sum fx}{\sum f} = \frac{2790}{40} = 69.75$

Using the values from the table above, $\sum f\lvert x - \bar{x}\rvert$ = 34.25 + 48.50 + 114 + 46.75 + 46 + 94.5 + 103 = 487

∴ Mean deviation $= \frac{\sum f\lvert x - \bar{x}\rvert}{\sum f}$

$= \frac{487}{40}$

∴ Mean deviation = 12.2

Practice Questions

1. Calculate the mean deviation of the following data: 0, 5, 7, 4, 5, 3

Solution

2. Calculate the mean deviation of the following data: 4, 6, 5, 9, 9, 5, 2, 4, 8, 6, 8

Solution

3. Calculate the mean deviation of the following data: 1, 3, 1, 4, 6

Solution

4. The marks obtained by 30 students in a physics test are as shown below. Calculate the mean deviation of the data.

Marks	0 - 9	10 - 19	20 - 29	30 - 39	40 - 49	50 - 59	60- 69
Number of student	4	1	5	8	3	2	7

Solution

5. The ages of 100 people in a village are as shown below. Calculate the mean deviation of the ages.

Age	11 - 20	21 - 30	31 - 40	41 - 50	51 - 60	61 - 70
Number of people	12	9	15	24	29	11

Solution

6. The number of employees in 50 enterprises are as shown below. Calculate the mean deviation of the data.

Marks	0 - 4	5 - 9	10 - 14	15 - 19	20 - 24	25 - 29	30- 34
Number of student	2	11	15	3	4	2	13

Solution

7. The table below shows the number of farms owned by some people in a city.

Number of farms	2	4	6	8	10	12
Number of people	3	5	10	6	8	8

Calculate the mean deviation of the data.

Solution

8. A die is rolled 50 times and the following data is obtained.

2	5	4	3	5	3	1	4	6	5	6	4	2
6	1	5	6	2	1	6	4	3	4	3	1	6
1	3	6	4	2	4	3	4	5	3	4	1	2
3	1	2	2	5	6	4	3	4	6	5		

(a) Present the data in a frequency table

(b) Calculate the mean deviation of the data.

Solution

(a)

(b)

Answers to Chapter 5

1. 1.67 2. 1.82 3. 1.6 4. 16.27 5. 12.5 6. 9.1 7. 2.7

8. (a) The frequency table is as shown below.

No on Die	1	2	3	4	5	6
No of Times	7	7	9	11	7	9

(b) 1.41

CHAPTER 6
VARIANCE AND STANDARD DEVIATION

Variance is the mean of the squares of the deviations from the mean. Standard deviation is the positive square root of the variance.

Variance, standard deviation and mean deviation are also regarded as measures of dispersion or variation.

The variance of data not given on a frequency table is given by:

$$\text{Variance} = \frac{\sum(x - \bar{x})^2}{\text{N}}$$

For data given on a frequency table, the variance is given by:

$$\text{Variance} = \frac{\sum \text{f}(x - \bar{x})^2}{\sum \text{f}}$$

Standard deviation is the square root of variance.

Examples

1. Calculate the variance and standard deviation of the following data: 4, 2, 1, 5.

Solution

Let us first calculate the mean of the data.

$$\text{Mean, } \bar{x} = \frac{4 + 2 + 1 + 5}{4} = \frac{12}{4} = 3$$

We now present the deviation from the mean as follows.

Data x	$x - \bar{x}$ $(\bar{x} = 3)$	$(x - \bar{x})^2$
4	1	1
2	-1	1
1	-2	4
5	2	4
		$\sum(x - \bar{x})^2 = 10$

$$\text{Variance} = \frac{\sum(x - \bar{x})^2}{\text{N}} = = \frac{10}{4} = 2.5$$

∴ Standard deviation = $\sqrt{2.5}$ = 1.58

2. The distances in Km, from school to the homes of 30 students are as shown below. Calculate:

(a) the variance
(b) the standard deviation of the data

Distance (Km)	0 - 4	5 - 9	10 – 14	15 - 19	20 - 24	25 - 29
Number of students	2	10	8	6	3	1

Solutions

The working is set out as shown on the table below

Distance	mid-value x	No of student f	fx	$x - \bar{x}$ $\bar{x} = 12.2$	$(x - \bar{x})^2$	$f(x - \bar{x})^2$
0 – 4	2	2	4	-10.2	104.04	208.08
5 – 9	7	10	70	-5.2	27.04	270.4
10 – 14	12	8	96	-0.2	0.04	0.32
15 – 19	17	6	102	4.8	23.04	138.24
20 – 24	22	3	66	9.8	96.04	288.12
25 – 29	27	1	27	14.8	219.04	219.04
		$\sum f = 30$	$\sum fx = 365$			

Mean, $\bar{x} = \frac{\sum fx}{\sum f} = \frac{365}{30} = 12.2$

(a) Using the values from the table above, $\sum f(x - \bar{x})^2 = 208.08 + 270.4 + 0.32 + 138.24 + 288.12 + 219.04 = 1124.2$

∴ Variance = $\frac{\sum f(x - \bar{x})^2}{\sum f}$

$= \frac{1124.2}{30}$

∴ Variance = 37.5

(b) Standard deviation = $\sqrt{\text{Variance}}$

$= \sqrt{37.5}$

∴ Standard deviation = 6.1

Practice Questions

1. Calculate the variance and standard deviation of the following data: 3, 5, 4, 7, 6.

Solution

2. Calculate the variance and standard deviation of the data below:
   1, 0, 4, 3, 5, 8, 6, 4, 7, 2.

Solution

3. The scores of 50 students in a test are as shown below. Calculate:

(a) the variance
(b) the standard deviation of the data

Scores	0 - 9	10 - 19	20 - 29	30 - 39	40 - 49	50 - 59
Number of students	5	12	6	18	5	4

Solution

(a)

(b)

4. The ages of employees in an organization are as shown below. Calculate:

(a) the variance
(b) the standard deviation of the data

Age	20 - 24	25 - 29	30 - 34	35 - 39	40 - 44
Number of empoyees	8	6	3	1	2

Solution

(a)

(b)

5. The scores obtained by 40 students in a test are as shown below. Calculate:

(a) the variance
(b) the standard deviation of the scores

Scores	5	6	7	8	9	10
Number of student	1	2	4	12	20	1

Solution

(a)

(b)

Answers to Chapter 6

1. Variance = 2	Standard Deviation = 1.41
2. Variance = 6	Standard Deviation = 2.45
3. (a) 199.04	(b) 14.11
4. (a) 40.69	(b) 6.38
5. (a) 1.049	(b) 1.024

Answers to Chapter 7

1. The frequency table is as shown below.

Mark	11 - 20	21 – 30	31 - 40	41 - 50	51 - 60	61 - 70	71 - 80	81 - 90	91-100
No of Student	4	5	4	5	8	3	5	3	3

(a) 53 (b) 33 (c) 72.5 (d) 39.5 (e) 19.75 (f) 38 (g) 64.5

2. (a) 32.36 (b) 25.18 (c) 40.25 (d) 15.07 (e) 7.54 (f) 41.6
(g) 37.33 (h) 22.06

3. (a) 1.7 (b) 1.23 (c) 2.31 (d) 1.60 (e) 0.98

4. (a) 17.5 (b) 11.29 (c) 22.56 (d) 11.27 (e) 5.63 (f) 20.06 (g) 29.5

5. (a) 1.54 (b) 0.83 (c) 2.08 (d) 0.83 (e) 1.01

CHAPTER 7
QUARTILES AND PERCENTILES BY INTERPOLATION METHOD

When a distribution is divide into four equal parts, it is called a quartile. When it is divided into hundred equal parts, such a division is called percentile.

The first quartile is also called lower quartile, and it is denoted by Q_1.
The second quartile is also called median, and it is denoted by Q_2.
The third quartile is also called upper quartile, and it is denoted by Q_3.

The lower quartile is calculated as follows:

$$Q_1 = L_1 + C\left(\frac{\frac{\Sigma f}{4} - CF_{bQ_1}}{F_{Q_1}}\right)$$

Where, $\frac{\Sigma f}{4}$ determines the lower quartile class
L_1 = Lower class boundary of the lower quartile class
CF_{bQ_1} = Cumulative frequency before the lower quartile class
F_{Q_1} = Frequency of the lower quartile class
C = Class width

The median is calculated as follows:

$$Q_2 = L_2 + C\left(\frac{\frac{\Sigma f}{2} - CF_{bm}}{F_m}\right)$$

Where, $\frac{\Sigma f}{2}$ determines the median class
L_2 = Lower class boundary of the median class
CF_{bm} = Cumulative frequency before the median class
F_m = Frequency of the median class
C = Class width

The upper quartile is calculated as follows:

$$Q_3 = L_3 + C\left(\frac{\frac{3\Sigma f}{4} - CF_{bQ_3}}{F_{Q_3}}\right)$$

Where, $\frac{3\sum f}{4}$ determines the upper quartile class

L_3 = Lower class boundary of the upper quartile class

CF_{bQ_3} = Cumulative frequency before the upper quartile class

F_{Q_3} = Frequency of the upper quartile class

C = Class width

The interquartile range is given by:

Interquartile range = $Q_3 - Q_1$

The semi-interquartile range is also called quartile deviation, and it is given by:

$$\text{Semi-interquartile range} = \frac{Q_3 - Q_1}{2}$$

The percentile is calculated as follows:

$$P_N = L_N + C\left(\frac{\frac{N\sum f}{100} - CF_{bP_N}}{F_{P_N}}\right)$$

Where P_N is the N percentile

Where, $\frac{N\sum f}{100}$ determines the N percentile class

L_N = Lower class boundary of the N percentile class

CF_{bP_N} = Cumulative frequency before the N percentile class

F_{P_N} = Frequency of the N percentile class

C = Class width

Example

The table below shows the distribution of marks scored by students in an examination.

Class interval	Frequency
60 – 64	2
65 – 69	4
70 – 74	7
75 – 79	13
80 – 84	10

85 – 89	8
90 – 94	5
95 – 99	1

From the data, calculate:

(a) median

(b) lower quartile

(c) upper quartile

(d) interquartile range

(e) semi-interquartile range

(f) 70th percentile

(g) the pass mark if 25% of the students passed

(h) the pass mark if it was later agreed that only 40% of the students should fail.

Solution

(a) In order to calculate the median, a table of the class boundaries and cumulative frequency has to be drawn as shown below.

Class interval	Class boundary	Frequency	Cumulative frequency	Class width
60 – 64	59.5 – 64.5	2	2	5
65 – 69	64.5 – 69.5	4	6	5
70 – 74	69.5 – 74.5	7	13	5
75 – 79	74.5 – 79.5	13	26	5
80 – 84	79.5 – 84.5	10	36	5
85 – 89	84.5 – 89.5	8	44	5
90 – 94	89.5 – 94.5	5	49	5
95 – 99	94.5 – 99.5	1	50	5

The median is calculated as follows:

$$Q_2 = L_2 + C\left(\frac{\frac{\Sigma f}{2} - CF_{bm}}{F_m}\right)$$

$\frac{\Sigma f}{2} = \frac{50}{2} = 25$. This shows that the median class is at the 25th position. This is the class, 75 – 79. This is obtained by looking at the cumulative frequency to see where the 25th position class falls.

L_2 = Lower class boundary of the median class = 74.5

CF_{bm} = Cumulative frequency before the median class = 13

F_m = Frequency of the median class. This is also 13

C = Class width = 5

$$\therefore \quad Q_2 = L_2 + C\left(\frac{\frac{\Sigma f}{2} - CF_{bm}}{F_m}\right)$$

$$= 74.5 + 5\left(\frac{\frac{50}{2} - 13}{13}\right)$$

$$= 74.5 + 5\left(\frac{25 - 13}{13}\right)$$

$$= 74.5 + 5\left(\frac{12}{13}\right)$$

$$= 74.5 + \left(\frac{5 \times 12}{13}\right)$$

$$= 74.5 + 4.6$$

$$Q_2 = 79.1$$

(b) The lower quartile is calculated as follows:

$$Q_1 = L_1 + C\left(\frac{\frac{\Sigma f}{4} - CF_{bQ_1}}{F_{Q_1}}\right)$$

$\frac{\Sigma f}{4} = \frac{50}{4} = 12.5$. Hence the lower quartile class is at the 12th or 13th position. This class is, 70 – 74.

L_1 = Lower class boundary of the lower quartile class = 69.5

CF_{bQ_1} = Cumulative frequency before the lower quartile class = 6

F_{Q_1} = Frequency of the lower quartile class = 7

C = Class width = 5

$$\therefore \quad Q_1 = L_1 + C\left(\frac{\frac{\Sigma f}{4} - CF_{bQ_1}}{F_{Q_1}}\right)$$

$$= 69.5 + 5\left(\frac{\frac{50}{4} - 6}{7}\right)$$

$$= 69.5 + 5\left(\frac{12.5 - 6}{7}\right)$$

$$= 69.5 + 5\left(\frac{6.5}{7}\right)$$

$$= 69.5 + \left(\frac{5 \times 6.5}{7}\right)$$

$$= 69.5 + 4.6$$

$$Q_1 = 74.1$$

(c) The upper quartile is calculated as follows:

$$Q_3 = L_3 + C\left(\frac{\frac{3\sum f}{4} - CF_{bQ3}}{F_{Q3}}\right)$$

$\frac{3\sum f}{4} = \frac{3 \times 50}{4} = 37.5$. Hence the upper quartile class is at the 37th or 38th position. This class is, 85 – 89.

L_3 = Lower class boundary of the upper quartile class = 84.5

CF_{bQ_3} = Cumulative frequency before the upper quartile class = 36

F_{Q_3} = Frequency of the upper quartile class = 8

C = Class width = 5

$$\therefore \quad Q_3 = L_3 + C\left(\frac{\frac{3\sum f}{4} - CF_{bQ3}}{F_{Q3}}\right)$$

$$= 84.5 + 5\left(\frac{\frac{3 \times 50}{4} - 36}{8}\right)$$

$$= 84.5 + 5\left(\frac{37.5 - 36}{8}\right)$$

$$= 84.5 + 5\left(\frac{1.5}{8}\right)$$

$$= 84.5 + 0.9$$

$$Q_3 = 85.4$$

(d) Interquartile range = $Q_3 - Q_1$

$= 85.4 - 74.1$

$= 11.3$

(e) Semi-interquartile range, $Q = \frac{Q_3 - Q_1}{2}$

$$= \frac{85.4 - 74.1}{2}$$

$$= \frac{11.3}{2}$$

$Q = 5.65$

(f) The 70th percentile is calculated as follows:

$$P_N = L_N + C\left(\frac{\frac{N\sum f}{100} - CF_{bP_N}}{F_{P_N}}\right)$$

$P_N = P_{70}$

$\frac{N\sum f}{100} = \frac{70 \text{ x } 50}{100} = 35$. Hence the 70th percentile class is at the 35th position. This class is: 80 - 84

$L_N = L_{70}$ = Lower class boundary of the 70th percentile class = 79.5

$CF_{bP_N} = CF_{bP_{70}}$ = Cumulative frequency before the 70th percentile class = 26

$F_{P_N} = F_{P_{70}}$ = Frequency of the 70th percentile class = 10

C = Class width = 5

Hence, $$P_{70} = L_{70} + C\left(\frac{\frac{70\sum f}{100} - CF_{bP_{70}}}{F_{P_{70}}}\right)$$

$$= 79.5 + 5\left(\frac{\frac{70 \text{ x } 50}{100} - 26}{10}\right)$$

$$= 79.5 + 5\left(\frac{35 - 26}{10}\right)$$

$$= 79.5 + 5\left(\frac{9}{10}\right)$$

$$= 79.5 + 4.5$$

$$P_{70} = 84$$

(g) If 25% of the students passed, then the first 75% (i.e. 100 – 25) of the students failed. This means that the pass mark is at the 75th percentile.

Note that the pass mark is always at the failure percentile.

Hence the 75th percentile is calculated as follows:

$$P_N = L_N + C\left(\frac{\frac{N\sum f}{100} - CF_{bP_N}}{F_{P_N}}\right)$$

$P_N = P_{75}$

$\frac{N\sum f}{100} = \frac{75 \text{ x } 50}{100} = 37.5$. Hence the 75th percentile class is at the 37.5th position. This class is: 85 - 89

$L_N = L_{75}$ = Lower class boundary of the 75th percentile class = 84.5

$CF_{bP_N} = CF_{bP_{75}}$ = Cumulative frequency before the 75th percentile class = 36
$F_{P_N} = F_{P_{75}}$ = Frequency of the 75th percentile class = 8
C = Class width = 5

Hence, $$P_{75} = L_{75} + C\left(\frac{\frac{75\sum f}{100} - CF_{bP_{75}}}{F_{P_{75}}}\right)$$

$$= 84.5 + 5\left(\frac{\frac{75 \times 50}{100} - 36}{8}\right)$$

$$= 84.5 + 5\left(\frac{37.5 - 36}{8}\right)$$

$$= 84.5 + 5\left(\frac{1.5}{8}\right)$$

$$= 84.5 + 0.9$$

$$P_{75} = 85.4$$

Hence the pass mark is 85.4

(h) If 40% of the students should fail, then the pass mark is at the 40th percentile.

Hence the 40th percentile is calculated as follows:

$$P_N = L_N + C\left(\frac{\frac{N\sum f}{100} - CF_{bP_N}}{F_{P_N}}\right)$$

$P_N = P_{40}$

$\frac{N\sum f}{100} = \frac{40 \times 50}{100}$ = 20. Hence the 40th percentile class is at the 20th position. This class is: 75 - 79
$L_N = L_{40}$ = Lower class boundary of the 40th percentile class = 74.5
$CF_{bP_N} = CF_{bP_{40}}$ = Cumulative frequency before the 40th percentile class = 13
$F_{P_N} = F_{P_{40}}$ = Frequency of the 40th percentile class = 13
C = Class width = 5

Hence, $$P_{40} = L_{40} + C\left(\frac{\frac{40\sum f}{100} - CF_{bP_{40}}}{F_{P_{40}}}\right)$$

$$= 74.5 + 5\left(\frac{\frac{40 \times 50}{100} - 13}{13}\right)$$

$$= 74.5 + 5\left(\frac{20 - 13}{13}\right)$$

$= 74.5 + 5(\frac{7}{13})$

$= 74.5 + 2.7$

$P_{40} = 77.2$

Hence the pass mark is 77.2

Practice Questions

1. The following is the record of marks of 40 students in an examination:

34 74 92 58 46 76 73 23 66 70 57 43 53 39
50 37 82 29 54 77 67 19 18 96 15 55 41 29
33 52 22 81 77 81 58 27 20 55 49 96

Using class interval 11 – 20, 21 – 30, ..., prepare a frequency table for the distribution.
Hence calculate the:
(a) median
(b) lower quartile
(c) upper quartile
(d) interquartile range
(e) quartile deviation/semi-interquartile range
(f) 30th percentile
(g) 68th percentile

Solution

(a)

(a)

(b)

(c)

(d)

(e)

(f)

(g)

2. The table below shows the distribution of marks scored by students in an examination.

Class interval	Frequency
10 – 14	1
15 – 19	3
20 – 24	8
25 – 29	11
30 – 34	7
35 – 39	9
40 – 44	10
45 – 49	5

From the data, calculate:

(a) median

(b) lower quartile

(c) upper quartile

(d) interquartile range

(e) semi-interquartile range

(f) 80th percentile

(g) the pass mark if 35% of the students passed

(h) the pass mark if 15% the students should fail.

Solution

(a)

(b)

(c)

(d)

(e)

(f)

(g)

(h)

3. The table below shows the height of some flowers sold in a farm.

Mass	0.5 – 0.9	1.0 – 1.4	1.5 – 1.9	2.0 – 2.4	2.5 – 2.9	3.0 – 3.4
No of Items	4	15	12	9	7	3

From the table given above, estimate:

(a) median
(b) lower quartile
(c) upper quartile
(d) the 45th percentile
(e) pass mark if 90% of the students passed

Solution

(a)

(b)

(c)

(d)

(e)

4. The table below shows the distribution of marks scored by students in an test.

Class interval	Frequency
0 – 4	1
5 – 9	4
10 – 14	7
15 – 19	5
20 – 24	9
25 – 29	1
30 – 34	2
35 – 39	1

From the data, calculate:

(a) median

(b) lower quartile

(c) upper quartile

(d) interquartile range

(e) semi-interquartile range

(f) 60th percentile

(g) the pass mark if 10% of the students passed

Solution

(a)

(b)

(c)

(d)

(e)

(f)

(g)

5. The table below shows the weight in gram of some seeds found in some cocoa pods.

Mass	0 – 0.4	0.5 – 0.9	1.0 – 1.4	1.5 – 1.9	2.0 – 2.4	2.5 – 2.9
No of Items	9	21	16	22	28	4

From the table given above, estimate:

(a) median
(b) lower quartile
(c) upper quartile
(d) the 25th percentile
(e) pass mark if 68% of the students passed

Solution

(a)

(b)

(c)

(d)

(e)

CHAPTER 8
THE BASIC THEORY OF PROBABILITY

Probability is the likelihood of an event happening. Mathematically probability is given by:

$$\text{Probability} = \frac{\text{number of required outcome}}{\text{number of total or possible outcome}}$$

If the probability of an event happening is x, then the probability that it will not happen will be given by:

$$1 - x$$

Probability must lie between the values of 0 and 1. If an event cannot happen, then its probably is 0. If an event is certain to happen, then its probability is 1.

Mutually Exclusive Events

When there is no member/element common between two or more similar events, then we say they are mutually exclusive events. For example the event of odd numbers or even numbers are mutually exclusive. They are disjoint sets.

Addition Law of Probability

If two events are mutually exclusive, then the probability of one or the other happening is the sum of their individual probabilities.

Independent Events

When a die is thrown, and a coin is tossed, these two events have no effect on each other. Such events are called independent events

Product law of probability

If two events are independent, then the probability of both events happening is the product is the product (multiplication) of their individual probabilities.

CHAPTER 9
PROBABILITY ON SIMPLE EVENTS

Examples

1. The table below give the number of students in each age group in a class.

Age (Years)	12	13	14	15	16	17
number of students	6	3	10	4	2	5

If a student is chosen at random, find the probability that the student is:
(a) 13 years old
(b) 15 years old or less
(c) at least 16 years old
(d) most 13 years old
(e) not 17 years old

Solution

(a) Pr. (13 years old) $= \frac{\text{Number of students who are 13 years old}}{\text{Total number of students}}$

$= \frac{3}{30}$

$= \frac{1}{10}$ (when $\frac{3}{30}$ is express in its lowest term, it gives $\frac{1}{10}$)

(b) Pr. (15 years or less) $= \frac{\text{Students who are 15 years and below}}{\text{Total number of students}}$

$= \frac{4+10+3+6}{30}$

$= \frac{23}{30}$

(c) Pr. (At least 16 years old) $= \frac{\text{Students who are 16 years and above}}{\text{Total number of students}}$

$= \frac{2+5}{30}$

$= \frac{7}{30}$

(d) Pr. (At most 13 years) $= \frac{\text{Students who are 13 years and below}}{\text{Total number of students}}$

$$= \frac{3+6}{30}$$

$$= \frac{9}{30}$$

$$= \frac{3}{10}$$ (When expressed in its lowest term)

(e) Pr. (17 years old) = $\frac{\text{number of students who are 17 years old}}{\text{total number of students}}$

$$= \frac{5}{30}$$

$$= \frac{1}{6}$$

Therefore, Pr. (Not 17 years old) = 1 - Pr. (17 years old)

$$= 1 - \frac{1}{6}$$

$$= \frac{5}{6}$$

2. The probability that a seed will germinate is $\frac{2}{5}$. What is the probability that it will not germinate?

Solution

Pr. (It will germinate) = $\frac{2}{5}$

Pr. (It will not germinate) = $1 - \frac{3}{5}$

$$= \frac{2}{5}$$

3. A letter is chosen at random from the alphabet. Find the probability that it is one of the letters of the word: PROBABILITY.

Solution

In this case a letter should not be counted more than once. Avoiding repetition, the word can now be written as:

PROBALITY (i.e. 9 letters). Note that there are 26 letters of the alphabet.

Therefore, Pr. (one letter from PROBABILITY) = $\frac{9}{26}$

4. A number is chosen at random between 1 and 16, both inclusive. What is the probability that it is:
(a) even
(b) prime
(c) odd or prime
(d) divisible by 4
(e) a perfect square or a perfect cube

Solution

(a) Total numbers in all from 1 to 16 = 16

The even numbers are 2, 4, 6, 8, 10, 12, 14, 16

Therefore the number of even numbers is 8

Hence Pr. (even number selected) = $\frac{\text{Number of even numbers}}{\text{Total numbers in all}}$

$= \frac{8}{16}$

$= \frac{1}{2}$

(b) The prime numbers are 2, 3, 5, 7, 11, 13

Therefore the number of prime numbers is 6

Hence Pr. (prime number selected) = $\frac{\text{Number of prime numbers}}{\text{Total numbers in all}}$

$= \frac{6}{16}$

$= \frac{3}{8}$

(c) The odd numbers are 1, 3, 5, 7, 9, 11, 13, 15

The prime numbers are 1, 3, 5, 7, 11, 13

Since OR in probability means addition, then we add all the odd and prime numbers together, but we must not count any number twice. This gives 1, 3, 5, 7, 9, 11, 13, 15, which is a total of 8 numbers.

Hence Pr. (odd or prime number selected) = $\frac{\text{Number of odd and even numbers}}{\text{Total numbers in all}}$

$= \frac{8}{16}$

$= \frac{1}{8}$

(d) The numbers divisible by 4 are 4, 8, 12, 16

This gives a total of 4 numbers

Hence Pr. (a number divisible by 4) = $\frac{\text{The four numbers divisible by 4}}{\text{Total numbers in all}}$

$= \frac{4}{16}$

$= \frac{1}{4}$

(e) The perfect square numbers are 1, 4, 9, 16

The perfect cube numbers are 1, 8

Since OR in probability means addition, then we add all the set of values above without counting any number twice. This gives 1, 4, 8, 9, 15, which is a total of 5 numbers.

Hence Pr. (perfect square or perfect cube selected) = $\frac{15}{16}$

5. A letter is chosen at random from the alphabet. Find the probability that it is:
(a) T
(b) E or P
(c) not B or G
(d) either D, J, N, U, W or Y
(e) one of the letters of the word REJECTED

Solution
(a) There are 26 letters of the alphabet, out of which there is 1 T.

Therefore, Pr. (T) = $\frac{\text{Number of Ts}}{\text{Total numbers of alphabets}}$

$$= \frac{1}{26}$$

(b) Pr. (E or P) = $\frac{\text{Number of Es and Ps}}{\text{Total numbers of alphabets}}$

$$= \frac{6}{26}$$

$$= \frac{1}{13}$$

(c) Pr. (B or G) = $\frac{2}{26} = \frac{1}{13}$

Therefore, Pr. (not B or G) = 1 - Pr. (B or G)

$$= 1 - (\frac{6}{13})$$

$$= \frac{12}{13}$$

(d) The letters D, J, N, U, W and Y makes a total of 6 letters.

Pr. (D, J, N, U, W or Y) = $\frac{6}{26}$

$$= \frac{3}{13}$$

(e) Writing the letters of the word REJECTED without repeating a letter gives REJCTD. This gives a total of 6 letters

Therefore Pr. (one of the letters of REJECTED) = $\frac{6}{26}$

$$= \frac{3}{13}$$

6. A letter is selected at random from the word PROBABILITY. What is the probability of selecting the letter B.

Solution

In this case the total letters of the word PROBABILITY gives 11. The repeated letters should be counted more than once since this is not a case of letter from the alphabet. In the 26 alphabet each letter appears once, that is why they are counted once. But in PROBABILITY (or other words that might be given) some letters appear more than once, hence they should be counted as many times as they appear.

In PROBABILITY, B appears 2 times.

Therefore, Pr. (selecting B) = $\frac{2}{11}$

Practice Questions

1. The table below give the number of students in each mark group in a class.

Mark	5	6	7	8	9	10
Number of students	3	6	2	4	1	4

If a student is chosen at random, find the probability that the student scored:
(a) 7 marks
(b) 6 marks or less
(c) at least 9 marks
(d) at most 8 marks
(e) 5 or 8 maks

Solution

(a)

(b)

(c)

(d)

(e)

2. The probability that a seed will germinate is $\frac{3}{4}$. What is the probability that it will not germinate?

Solution

3. A letter is chosen at random from the alphabet. Find the probability that it is one of the letters of the word: MATHEMATICS.

Solution

4. The probability that a man wins an election is $\frac{3}{5}$. What is the probability that he does not win.

Solution

5. Out of every 10 bulbs, 2 do not last long. What is the probability that a bulb will last long when lit?

Solution

6. In family, the number of males is 3, while the number of females is 2. Find the probability that another child born into the family is:
(a) a male child
(b) a female child

Solution

(a)

(b)

7. A survey shows that 44% of all women take size 7 shoes. What is the probability that a mother of two takes size 7 shoes?

Solution

8. In a secondary school, 30 out of every 100 students are at least 160cm tall. What is the probability that a student chosen at random from the school is less than 160cm tall?

Solution

9. A number is chosen at random between 1 and 20, both inclusive. What is the probability that it is:
(a) prime
(b) odd

(c) even or prime
(d) divisible by 3
(e) a number less than 10 or a perfect cube

Solution

(a)

(b)

(c)

(d)

(e)

10. A letter is chosen at random from the alphabet. Find the probability that it is:
(a) F
(b) M or Q or Y
(c) in the word COME
(d) either in the word BUT or in REMOVE
(e) one of the letters of the word SURPRISED

Solution

(a)

(b)

(c)

(d)

(e)

11. A letter is selected at random from the word RESPIRATION. What is the probability of selecting the letter I.

Solution

Answers to Chapter 9

1. (a) $\frac{1}{10}$ (b) $\frac{9}{20}$ (c) $\frac{1}{4}$ (d) $\frac{3}{4}$ (e) $\frac{7}{20}$

2. $\frac{1}{4}$ 3. $\frac{4}{13}$ 4. $\frac{2}{5}$ 5. $\frac{4}{5}$

6. (a) $\frac{3}{5}$ (b) $\frac{2}{5}$

7. $\frac{11}{25}$ 8. $\frac{7}{10}$

9. (a) $\frac{2}{5}$ (b) $\frac{1}{2}$ (c) $\frac{9}{10}$ (d) $\frac{3}{10}$ (e) $\frac{9}{20}$

10. (a) $\frac{1}{26}$ (b) $\frac{3}{26}$ (c) $\frac{2}{13}$ (d) $\frac{4}{13}$ (e) $\frac{4}{13}$

11. $\frac{2}{11}$

CHAPTER 10
PROBABILITY ON PACK OF PLAYING CARDS

A pack of playing cards contains 52 cards of 4 types. There are 13 clubs, 13 diamonds, 13 hearts and 13 spades. Each of the set of 13 cards contains Ace (A), 2, 3, 4, 5, 6, 7, 8, 9, 10, Jack (J), Queen (Q), and King (K). This means that out of the 52 cards, each card is four in number, i.e. Aces are 4 in number, 1s are 4 in number, 2s are 4 in number, 3s are 4 in number, 4s are 4 in number, 5s are 4 in number, 6s are 4 in number, 7s are 4 in number, 8s are 4 in number, 9s are 4 in number, 10s are 4 in number, Jacks are 4 in number, Queens are 4 in number, and Kings are 4 in number. Clubs and spades are black, diamonds and hearts are red. This means that there are 26 black cards and 26 red cards. This also means that out of the 4 Aces cards, 2 are black and 2 are red. Out of the four cards that are 1s, two are black and two are red, out of the four cards that are 2, two are black and two are red, and so on.

Examples

1. A card is picked at random from a pack of playing cards. Find the probability of picking a spade.

Solution

There are 13 spades in a pack of playing cards.

Therefore, Pr. (picking a spade) = $\frac{\text{Number of Spades}}{\text{Total numbers of cards}}$

$= \frac{13}{52}$

$= \frac{1}{4}$ (In its lowest term)

2. A card is picked at random from a pack of playing cards. Find the probability of picking a red card.

Solution

There are 26 red cards in a pack of playing cards.

Therefore, Pr. (picking a red card) = $\frac{\text{Number of red cards}}{\text{Total numbers of cards}}$

$= \frac{26}{52}$

$= \frac{1}{2}$ (In its lowest term)

3. A card is picked at random from a pack of playing cards. Find the probability of picking a red 5.

Solution

There are 2 red 5 cards in a pack of playing cards.

Therefore, Pr. (picking a red 5) = $\frac{\text{Number of red 5}}{\text{Total numbers of cards}}$

$= \frac{2}{52}$

$= \frac{1}{26}$ (In its lowest term)

4. A card is picked at random from a pack of playing cards. Find the probability of picking a 3.

Solution

There are 4 cards that are 3 in a pack of playing cards.

Therefore, Pr. (picking a 3) = $\frac{\text{Number of cards that are 3}}{\text{Total numbers of cards}}$

$= \frac{4}{52}$

$= \frac{1}{13}$ (In its lowest term)

5. A card is picked at random from a pack of playing cards. Find the probability of picking

(a) a black or red card

(b) a 2 or a 5

(c) either a heart or the king of spades

(d) a club or a red Queen

(e) a diamond or a 9

(f) a 6 or a black card

Solution

(a) There are 26 black cards and 26 red card

Since or in probability means plus, then we have to add the numbers. This gives a total of: 26 + 26 = 52

Therefore, Pr. (picking a black or red card) = $\frac{\text{Number of black and red cards}}{\text{Total numbers of cards}}$

$= \frac{52}{52}$

= 1

(b) There are 4 cards that are 2, and 4 cards that are 5. This gives a total of 8 cards.

Therefore, Pr. (picking a 2 or a 5) = $\frac{8}{52}$

$= \frac{2}{13}$

(c) There are 13 cards that are Hearts, and 1 king that is a spade. This gives a total of 14 cards.

Therefore, Pr. (picking either a heart or the king of spades) = $\frac{14}{52}$

$= \frac{7}{26}$

(d) There are 13 cards that are club, and 2 cards that are red Queen, (i.e. the Queen of hearts and the queen of diamond). This gives a total of 15 cards.

Therefore, Pr. (picking a club or a red Queen) = $\frac{15}{52}$

(e) There are 13 cards that are diamonds, and 4 cards that are 9. But one of the 9 is in diamond and has already been counted among the 13 diamonds. So it must not be counted twice. Hence we count the other three 9 (each from clubs, hearts and spades). This will give a total of 16 (13 + 3) cards.

Therefore, Pr. (picking a diamond or a 9) = $\frac{16}{52}$

$= \frac{4}{13}$

(f) There are 4 cards that are 6, and 26 cards that are black. But two of the 26 black cards are among the four cards that are 6, and these two black 6 cards have already been counted among the 26 black cards. So they must not be counted twice. Hence we count the other two 6 cards that are red. This will give a total of 28 (26 + 2) cards.

Therefore, Pr. (picking a 6 or a back card) = $\frac{28}{52}$

$= \frac{7}{13}$

6. A card is picked at random from a pack of playing cards and then replaced. A second card is picked. What is the probability of picking:

(a) a 3 and a 10

(b) a queen and an ace

(c) two kings

(d) two red cards

(e) two cards of different colour

(f) two cards of the same colours

Solution

In probability problems, when two items are selected, it is important to logically analyse the situation when solving the problem. This will help you to know if addition (use of OR) is involved or multiplication (use of AND) is involved. For example, for a queen and a king to be selected, it simply means that, either the queen is selected first and then the king, or the king is selected first and then the queen. When this logical analysis is understood, then most questions in probability become easy to solve.

(a) There are four cards that are 3, and four cards that are 10

Therefore, Pr. (picking a 3) = $\frac{4}{52}$

$= \frac{1}{13}$

Similarly, Pr. (picking a 10) = $\frac{4}{52}$

$= \frac{1}{13}$

Recall that "and" in probability means multiplication.

The probability of picking a 3 and a 10 means that:

Either the first is a 3 AND the second is a 10, OR the first is a 10 AND the second is a 3.

This can be calculated by putting x in place of AND and + in place of OR in the above statement as follows:

Pr. (picking a 3) x Pr. (picking a 10) + Pr. (picking a 10) x Pr. (picking a 3)

$$= (\frac{1}{13} \times \frac{1}{13}) + (\frac{1}{13} \times \frac{1}{13})$$

$$= \frac{1}{169} + \frac{1}{169}$$

$$= \frac{2}{169}$$

Therefore, Pr. (picking a 3 and a 10) = $\frac{2}{169}$

(b) There are 4 cards that are queen, and 4 cards that are ace

Therefore, Pr. (picking a queen) = $\frac{4}{52}$

$$= \frac{1}{13}$$

Similarly, Pr. (picking an ace) = $\frac{4}{52}$

$$= \frac{1}{13}$$

The probability of picking a queen and an ace means that:

Either you first pick a queen AND then an ace, OR you first pick an ace AND then a queen.

This can be calculated by putting x in place of AND and + in place of OR in the above statement as follows:

Pr. (picking a queen) x Pr. (picking an ace) + Pr. (picking an ace) x Pr. (picking a queen)

$$= (\frac{1}{13} \times \frac{1}{13}) + (\frac{1}{13} \times \frac{1}{13})$$

$$= \frac{1}{169} + \frac{1}{169}$$

$$= \frac{1}{169}$$

Therefore, Pr. (picking a queen and an ace) = $\frac{2}{169}$

(c) There are four cards that are King

Therefore, Pr. (picking a king) = $\frac{4}{52}$

$= \frac{1}{13}$

The probability of picking two kings means that:

The first is a king AND the second is a king

= Pr. (picking a king) x Pr. (picking a king)

$= \frac{1}{13} \times \frac{1}{13}$

$= \frac{1}{169}$

Therefore, Pr. (picking two kings) = $\frac{1}{169}$

(d) There are 26 cards that are red

Therefore, Pr. (picking a red card) = $\frac{26}{52}$

$= \frac{1}{2}$

The probability of picking two red cards means that:

The first is a red card AND the second is a red card

= Pr. (picking a red card) x Pr. (picking a red card)

$= \frac{1}{2} \times \frac{1}{2}$

$= \frac{1}{4}$

Therefore, Pr. (picking two red cards) = $\frac{1}{4}$

(e) There are two colours of cards, red and black.

Therefore, Pr. (picking a red card) = $\frac{1}{2}$ (i.e from $\frac{26}{52}$ since there are 26 red cards)

Similarly, Pr. (picking a black card) = $\frac{1}{2}$ (i.e from $\frac{26}{52}$ since there are also 26 black cards)

The probability of picking two cards of different colours means that:

Either the first is a black card AND the second is a red card, OR the first is a red card AND the second is a black card.

This can be calculated by putting x in place of AND and + in place of OR in the above statement as follows:

Pr. (picking a black card) x Pr. (picking a red card) + Pr. (picking a red card) x Pr. (picking a black card)

$$= (\frac{1}{2} \times \frac{1}{2}) + (\frac{1}{2} \times \frac{1}{2})$$

$$= \frac{1}{4} + \frac{1}{4}$$

$$= \frac{2}{4}$$

$$= \frac{1}{2}$$

Therefore, Pr. (picking two cards of different colours) = $\frac{1}{2}$

(f) Pr. (picking two cards of the same colours) = 1 - Pr. (picking two cards of different colours)

$$= 1 - \frac{1}{2}$$

$$= \frac{1}{2}$$

Note that this can also be solved by using the logical process which is:

Either the first is red AND the second is red OR the first is black AND the second is black. This will also give $\frac{1}{2}$

7. Two cards are picked at random one after the other without replacement from a pack of playing cards. What is the probability of picking:

(a) a 5 and a 7

(b) a king and a jack

(c) two aces

(d) two diamond cards
(e) two black cards
(f) a red and a black card
(g) two cards of the same colours

Solution

This problem involves picking a card without replacement. This means that when one card is picked out, the total number of cards remaining in the pack become reduced to 51. That number of that particular type of card also reduces by 1.

(a) There are four cards that are 5. There are also four cards that are 7.

Hence the probability of picking a 5 and a 7 means that:

Either first picking a 5 AND then a 7, OR first picking a 7 AND then a 5.

Now, let us calculate each of the probabilities as follows:

Pr. (first card is a 5) = $\frac{4}{52}$ (There are four cards that are 5)

= $\frac{1}{13}$ (In its lowest term)

We now have 51 cards left in the pack.

Therefore, Pr. (second card is a 7) = $\frac{4}{51}$ (There are four cards that are 7, and a total of 51 cards remaining in the pack)

Or,

Pr. (first card is a 7) = $\frac{4}{52}$ (There are four cards that are 7)

= $\frac{1}{13}$ (In its lowest term)

We now have 51 cards left in the pack.

Therefore, Pr. (second card is a 5) = $\frac{4}{51}$ (There are four cards that are 5, and a total of 51 cards remaining in the pack)

Hence the probability of picking a 5 and a 7 means that:

Either first picking a 5 AND then a 7, OR first picking a 7 AND then a 5. Which is computed as:

Pr. (picking a 5 and a 7) = Pr. (first card is a 5) x Pr. (second card is a 7) + Pr. (first card is a 7) x Pr. (second card is a 5)

$$= (\frac{1}{13} \times \frac{4}{51}) + (\frac{1}{13} \times \frac{4}{51})$$

$$= \frac{4}{663} + \frac{4}{663}$$

$$= \frac{8}{663}$$

(b) There are four cards that are kings. There are also four cards that are jacks.

Now, let us calculate each of the probabilities as follows:

Pr. (first card is a king) = $\frac{4}{52}$ (There are four cards that are kings)

$= \frac{1}{13}$ (In its lowest term)

We now have 51 cards left in the pack.

Therefore, Pr. (second card is a jack) = $\frac{4}{51}$ (There are four cards that are jack, and a total of 51 cards remaining in the pack)

Or,

Pr. (first card is a jack) = $\frac{4}{52}$ (There are four cards that are jack)

$= \frac{1}{13}$ (In its lowest term)

We now have 51 cards left in the pack.

Therefore, Pr. (second card is a king) = $\frac{4}{51}$ (There are four cards that are king, and a total of 51 cards remaining in the pack)

Hence the probability of picking a king and a jack means that:

Either first picking a king AND then a jack, OR first picking a jack AND then a king. This is computed as:

Pr. (picking a king and a queen) = Pr. (first card is a king) x Pr. (second card is a jack) + Pr. (first card is a jack) x Pr. (second card is a king)

$$= \left(\frac{1}{13} \times \frac{4}{51}\right) + \left(\frac{1}{13} \times \frac{4}{51}\right)$$

$$= \frac{4}{663} + \frac{4}{663}$$

$$= \frac{8}{663}$$

(c) There are 4 cards that are aces.

Hence the probability of picking two aces means that:

The first is an ace, and the second is an ace.

Now, let us calculate each of the probabilities as follows:

Pr. (first card is an ace) = $\frac{4}{52}$ (There are 4 cards that are aces)

$= \frac{1}{13}$ (In its lowest term)

We now have 3 aces left in the pack, and a total of 51 cards left in the pack.

Therefore, Pr. (second card is an ace) = $\frac{3}{51}$

Hence the probability of picking two aces is given by:

Pr. (picking two aces) = Pr. (first card is an ace) x Pr. (second card is an ace)

$$= \frac{1}{13} \times \frac{3}{51}$$

$$= \frac{3}{663}$$

(d) There are 13 cards that are diamonds.

Hence the probability of picking two diamonds means that:

The first is a diamond, and the second is a diamond.

Now, let us calculate each of the probabilities as follows:

Pr. (first card is a diamond) = $\frac{13}{52}$ (There are 13 cards that are diamonds)

$= \frac{1}{4}$ (In its lowest term)

We now have 12 diamonds left in the pack, and a total of 51 cards left in the pack.

Therefore, Pr. (second card is a diamond) = $\frac{1}{13}$

$= \frac{4}{17}$ (In its lowest term)

Hence the probability of picking two diamonds is given by:

Pr. (picking two diamonds) = Pr. (first card is a diamond) x Pr. (second card is a diamond)

$= \frac{1}{4} \text{ x } \frac{4}{17}$

$= \frac{4}{68}$

$= \frac{1}{17}$ (In its lowest term)

(e) There are 26 black cards.

Hence the probability of picking two black cards means that:

The first is a black card, and the second is a black card.

Now, let us calculate each of the probabilities as follows:

Pr. (first card is a black card) = $\frac{26}{52}$

$= \frac{1}{2}$ (In its lowest term)

We now have 25 black cards left in the pack, and a total of 51 cards left in the pack.

Therefore, Pr. (second card is a black card) = $\frac{25}{51}$

Hence the probability of picking two black cards is given by:

Pr. (picking two black cards) = Pr. (first card is a black card) x Pr. (second card is a black card)

$$= \frac{1}{2} \times \frac{25}{51}$$

$$= \frac{25}{102}$$

(f) The logical explanation for this situation is that:

Either the first card is red AND the second is black OR the first card is black and the second is red.

There are 26 red cards and also 26 black cards.

Now, let us calculate each of the probabilities as follows:

Pr. (first card is a red card) = $\frac{26}{52}$

$= \frac{1}{2}$ (In its lowest term)

We now have 51 cards left in the pack.

Therefore, Pr. (second card is a black card) = $\frac{26}{51}$ (There are 26 black cards, and a total of 51 cards remaining in the pack)

Or,

Pr. (first card is a black card) = $\frac{26}{52}$

$= \frac{1}{2}$ (In its lowest term)

We now have 51 cards left in the pack.

Therefore, Pr. (second card is a red card) = $\frac{26}{51}$ (There are 26 red cards, and a total of 51 cards remaining in the pack)

Hence the probability of picking a red card and a black card means that:

Either first picking a red card AND then a black card, OR first picking a black card AND then a red card. This is computed as:

Pr. (picking a red and black cards) = Pr. (first card is a red card) x Pr. (second card is a black card) + Pr. (first card is a black card) x Pr. (second card is a red card)

$$= (\frac{1}{2} x \frac{26}{51}) + (\frac{1}{2} x \frac{26}{51})$$

$$= \frac{26}{102} + \frac{26}{102}$$

$$= \frac{52}{102}$$

$$= \frac{26}{51}$$

(g) The logical explanation for this situation is that:

Either the first card is red AND the second is red OR the first card is black and the second is black.

There are 26 red cards and also 26 black cards.

Now, let us calculate each of the probabilities as follows:

Pr. (first card is a red card) = $\frac{26}{52}$

$= \frac{1}{2}$ (In its lowest term)

We now have 25 red cards left and a total of 51 cards left in the pack.

Therefore, Pr. (second card is a red card) = $\frac{25}{51}$

Or,

Pr. (first card is a black card) = $\frac{26}{102}$

$= \frac{1}{2}$ (In its lowest term)

We now have 25 black cards left and a total of 51 cards left in the pack.

Therefore, Pr. (second card is a black card) = $\frac{25}{51}$

Hence the probability of picking two cards of the same colour means that:

Either picking a red card AND then another red card, OR picking a black card AND then another black card. Which is computed as:

Pr. (picking two cards of the same colour) = Pr. (first card is a red card) x Pr. (second card is a red card) + Pr. (first card is a black card) x Pr. (second card is a black card)

$$= (\frac{1}{2} \times \frac{25}{51}) + (\frac{1}{2} \times \frac{25}{51})$$

$$= \frac{25}{102} + \frac{25}{102}$$

$$= \frac{50}{102}$$

$$= \frac{25}{51}$$

Alternatively, this question can also be solved as follows:

Recall that question (f) above gives the probability of picking a red and a black card. This also means the probability of picking two cards of different colours.

Hence the probability of picking two cards of different colours as given in (f) above = $\frac{26}{51}$

Therefore, Pr. (picking two cards of the same colour) = 1 - Pr. (picking two cards of different colours) (Note that they are opposite statements)

$$= 1 - \frac{26}{51}$$

$$= \frac{51-26}{51}$$

$$= \frac{25}{51} \quad \text{(As obtained before)}$$

8. If three cards are chosen from a pack of playing cards without replacement, what is the probability of getting:
(a) at least two diamonds
(b) at most one diamond?

Solution

Now, in order to write out the outcomes, let us use the letter D to represent a diamond and letter N to represent not a diamond.

Hence the outcomes are written as follows:

(DDD), (DDN), (DND), (DNN), (NDD), (NDN), (NND), (NNN)

(a) In order to determine the probability of getting at least two diamonds, we need to compute the probabilities of the brackets that contain at least 2 diamonds. They are, (DDD), (DDN), (DND), and (NDD).

Hence the probability of getting at least two diamonds = (DDD) or (DDN) or (DND) or (NDD)

Now, let us compute each of the probabilities.

There are 13 diamonds in a pack of cards, and there are 39 cards that are not diamonds. Note that this is a case of without replacement, which means that after each selection, both the total number of cards left and the number of the particular card picked, are reduced by 1. Hence:

(DDD) = Pr. (first card is a diamond) x Pr. (second card is a diamond) x Pr. (third card is a diamond)

$= \frac{13}{52} \text{X} \frac{12}{51} \text{X} \frac{11}{50}$ (Note that the number of diamond and the total number of card left, keep reducing by 1 after each selection)

$= \frac{1}{4} \text{X} \frac{12}{51} \text{X} \frac{11}{50}$

$= \frac{132}{10200}$

$= \frac{11}{850}$ (In its lowest term, after equal division by 12)

(DDN) = Pr. (first card is a diamond) x Pr. (second card is a diamond) x Pr. (third card is not a diamond)

$= \frac{13}{52} \text{X} \frac{12}{51} \text{X} \frac{39}{50}$ (Note that there are 39 cards that are not diamond)

$= \frac{1}{4} \text{X} \frac{4}{17} \text{X} \frac{39}{50}$

$= \frac{156}{3400}$

$= \frac{39}{850}$ (After equal division by 4)

(DND) = Pr. (first card is a diamond) x Pr. (second card is not a diamond) x Pr. (third card is a diamond)

$= \frac{13}{52} \text{X} \frac{39}{51} \text{X} \frac{12}{50}$

$= \frac{1}{4} \text{ X } \frac{13}{17} \text{ X } \frac{6}{25}$

$= \frac{78}{1700}$

$= \frac{39}{850}$

(NDD) = Pr. (first card is not a diamond) x Pr. (second card is a diamond) x Pr. (third card is a diamond)

$= \frac{39}{52} \text{ X } \frac{13}{51} \text{ X } \frac{12}{50}$

$= \frac{3}{4} \text{ X } \frac{13}{51} \text{ X } \frac{6}{25}$

$= \frac{234}{5100}$

$= \frac{39}{850}$

Therefore, Pr. (getting at least two diamonds) = (DDD) or (DDN) or (DND) or (NDD)

= (DDD) + (DDN) + (DND) + (NDD)

$= \frac{11}{850} + \frac{39}{850} + \frac{39}{850} + \frac{39}{850}$

$= \frac{128}{850}$

$= \frac{64}{425}$

(b) In order to determine the probability of getting at most one diamond, we need to compute the probabilities of the brackets that contain at most one diamond. From the outcome brackets given above, the ones that contain at most one diamond are, (DNN), (NDN), (NND), (NNN). Note that at most one, means one and below, (i.e. one and zero diamond in this case).

Hence the probability of getting at most one diamond = (DNN) + (NDN) + (NND) + (NNN)

Now, let us compute each of the probabilities. Hence:

(DNN) = Pr. (first card is a diamond) x Pr. (second card is not a diamond) x Pr. (third card is not a diamond)

$= \frac{13}{52} \text{ X } \frac{39}{51} \text{ X } \frac{38}{50}$

$= \frac{1}{4} \text{ x } \frac{13}{17} \text{ x } \frac{19}{25}$

$= \frac{247}{1700}$

(NDN) = Pr. (first card is not a diamond) x Pr. (second card is a diamond) x Pr. (third card is not a diamond)

$= \frac{39}{52} \text{ x } \frac{13}{51} \text{ x } \frac{38}{50}$

$= \frac{3}{4} \text{ x } \frac{13}{51} \text{ x } \frac{19}{25}$

$= \frac{741}{5100}$

$= \frac{247}{1700}$ (In its lowest term after equal division by 3)

(NND) = Pr. (first card is not a diamond) x Pr. (second card is not a diamond) x Pr. (third card is a diamond)

$= \frac{39}{52} \text{ x } \frac{38}{51} \text{ x } \frac{13}{50}$

$= \frac{3}{4} \text{ x } \frac{38}{51} \text{ x } \frac{13}{50}$

$= \frac{1482}{10200}$

$= \frac{247}{1700}$ (After equal division by 6)

(NNN) = Pr. (first card is not a diamond) x Pr. (second card is not a diamond) x Pr. (third card is not a diamond)

$= \frac{39}{52} \text{ x } \frac{38}{51} \text{ x } \frac{37}{50}$

$= \frac{3}{4} \text{ x } \frac{38}{51} \text{ x } \frac{37}{50}$

$= \frac{4218}{10200}$

$= \frac{703}{1700}$ (After equal division by 6)

Therefore, Pr. (getting at most one diamond) = (DNN) or (NDN) or (NND) or (NNN)

= (DNN) + (NDN) + (NND) + (NNN)

$$= \frac{247}{1700} + \frac{247}{1700} + \frac{247}{1700} + \frac{703}{1700}$$

$$= \frac{1444}{1700}$$

$$= \frac{361}{425}$$

Practice Questions

1. A card is picked at random from a pack of playing cards. Find the probability of picking a jack.

Solution

2. A card is picked at random from a pack of playing cards. Find the probability of picking a black 4.

Solution

3. A card is picked at random from a pack of playing cards. Find the probability of picking a red king.

Solution

4. A card is picked at random from a pack of playing cards. Find the probability of picking a either a black or red card.

Solution

5. A card is picked at random from a pack of playing cards. Find the probability of picking a black Queen.

Solution

6. A card is picked at random from a pack of playing cards. Find the probability of picking a card that is not an Ace.

Solution

7. A card is picked at random from a pack of playing cards. Find the probability of picking
(a) a queen or a king
(b) a 3 or a 9
(c) either a jack or the queen of diamonds
(d) a spade or a black 7
(e) a club or a red king
(f) a 2 or a red card

Solution

(a)

(c)

(d)

(e)

(f)

8. A card is picked at random from a pack of playing cards and then replaced. A second card is picked. What is the probability of picking:

(a) an 8 and a 5

(b) a black card and a 4

(c) two cards between 2 and 9 that have odd numbers

(d) two black cards

(e) two cards with the same number on them

(f) two cards with different number on them

Solution

(a)

(b)

(c)

(d)

(e)

(f)

9. Two cards are picked at random one after the other without replacement from a pack of playing cards. What is the probability of picking:

(a) a 4 and an ace

(b) a 2 and a 7

(c) two 8s

(d) two clubs

(e) two red cards

(f) a club and a diamond

(g) two cards that are queens

Solution

(a)

(b)

(c)

(d)

(e)

(f)

(g)

10. If three cards are picked from a pack of playing cards with replacement, what is the probability if getting:

(a) at least two 9s

(b) at most two 9s

Solution

(a)

(b)

11. If three cards are chosen from a pack of playing cards without replacement, what is the probability of getting:
(a) at least two kings
(b) at most one king?

Solution

(a)

(b)

Answers to Chapter 10

1. $\frac{1}{13}$ 2. $\frac{1}{26}$ 3. $\frac{1}{26}$ 4. 1 5. $\frac{1}{26}$ 6. $\frac{12}{13}$

7. (a) $\frac{2}{13}$ (b) $\frac{2}{13}$ (c) $\frac{5}{52}$ (d) $\frac{7}{26}$ (e) $\frac{15}{52}$ (f) $\frac{7}{13}$

8. (a) $\frac{1}{169}$ (b) $\frac{1}{13}$ (c) $\frac{6}{169}$ (d) $\frac{1}{4}$ (e) $\frac{1}{13}$ (f) $\frac{12}{13}$

9. (a) $\frac{8}{663}$ (b) $\frac{8}{663}$ (c) $\frac{1}{221}$ (d) $\frac{1}{17}$ (e) $\frac{25}{102}$ (f) $\frac{13}{102}$ (g) $\frac{1}{221}$

10. (a) $\frac{37}{2197}$ (b) $\frac{2196}{2197}$

11. (a) $\frac{73}{5525}$ (b) $\frac{5452}{5525}$

CHAPTER 11
PROBABILITY ON TOSSING OF COINS

When a coin is tossed, the outcome can either be a head or a tail. However when two or more coins are tossed, the total outcome is obtained from 2^n, where n is the number of times the coin is tossed, or the number of coins tossed together.

Note that 'head' is the part of the coin that shows the person drawn on the coin, while the opposite side of the coin is called the 'tail'

Examples

1. A fair coin is tossed. What is the probability of getting:
(a) a head
(b) a tail

Solution
(a) There are only two possible outcomes. Head or tail.

Therefore, Pr. (getting a head) = $\frac{\text{Number of heads}}{\text{Total outcomes}}$

$= \frac{1}{2}$

(b) Pr. (getting a tail) = $\frac{\text{Number of tails}}{\text{Total outcomes}}$

$= \frac{1}{2}$

2. A coin is tossed two times. What is the probability of getting:
(a) a head and a tail
(b) at least a tail
(c) two heads
(d) two tails
(e) a head on the first toss, and a tail on the second toss.

Solution
The outcomes are written by using H for head and T for tail. The total number of outcomes will be 2^2 = 4 (i.e. from 2^n, and n = 2 in this case)

The outcomes are: (HH), (HT), (TH), (TT).

(a) The outcomes with head and tail are (HT) and (TH). This gives 2 outcomes.

Therefore, Pr. (getting a head and tail) = $\frac{\text{Number of outcome with head and tail}}{\text{Total outcomes}}$

$= \frac{2}{4}$

$= \frac{1}{2}$

(b) The outcomes with at least a tail are (HT), (TH) and (TT). This gives 3 outcomes.

Therefore, Pr. (getting at least a tail) = $\frac{\text{Number of outcomes with at least a tail}}{\text{Total number of outcomes}}$

$= \frac{3}{4}$

(c) The outcome with two heads is (HH). This gives 1 outcome.

Therefore, Pr. (getting two heads) = $\frac{\text{Number of outcomes with heads}}{\text{Total number of outcomes}}$

$= \frac{1}{4}$

(d) The outcome with two tails is (TT). This gives 1 outcome.

Therefore, Pr. (getting two tails) = $\frac{\text{Number of outcomes with two tails}}{\text{Total number of outcomes}}$

$= \frac{1}{4}$

(e) The outcome with a head on the first toss, and a tail on the second toss is (HT). This gives 1 outcome

Therefore, Pr. (getting a head on the first toss, and a tail on the second toss) = $\frac{1}{4}$

3. A coin is tossed three times. What is the probability of getting:
(a) two heads and one tail
(b) at least one head
(c) three tails

(d) at least two heads
(e) a tail, a head and a tail

Solution

(a) The total number of outcomes will be $2^3 = 8$ (i.e. from 2^n, and n = 3 in this case)

The outcomes are: (HHH), (HTH), (HTT), (HHT), (THH), (THT), (TTH), (TTT). This gives a total of 8 outcomes

The outcomes with two heads and one tail are (HTH), (HHT) and (THH). This gives 3 outcomes.

Therefore, Pr. (getting two heads and one tail) = $\frac{\text{Number of outcomes with two heads and one tail}}{\text{Total number of outcomes}}$

$= \frac{3}{8}$

(b) The outcomes with at least one head are (HHH), (HTH), (HTT), (HHT), (THH), (THT) and (TTH). This gives 7 outcomes.

Therefore, Pr. (getting at least one head) = $\frac{\text{Number of outcomes with at least one head}}{\text{Total number of outcomes}}$

$= \frac{7}{8}$

(c) The outcome with three tails is (TTT). This gives 1 outcome.

Therefore, Pr. (getting three tails) = $\frac{1}{8}$

(d) The outcomes with at least two heads are (HHH), (HTH), (HHT) and (THH). This gives 4 outcomes.

Therefore, Pr. (getting at least two heads) = $\frac{\text{Number of outcomes with at least two heads}}{\text{Total number of outcomes}}$

$= \frac{4}{8}$

$= \frac{1}{2}$

(e) The outcome with a tail, a head and a tail is (THT). This is 1 outcome

Hence, Pr. (getting a tail, a head and a tail) = $\frac{1}{8}$

4. Four coins are tossed together. Find the probability of getting:
(a) two heads and two tails
(b) four tails
(c) at least three heads
(d) at least two heads
(e) one head

Solution

The total number of outcomes will be $2^4 = 16$ (i.e. from 2^n, and n = 4 in this case)

The outcomes are: (HHHH), (HHHT), (HHTT), (HTTT), (THHH), (TTHH), (TTTH), (THTH), (HTHT), (HHTH), (THHT), HTTH), (TTHT), (THTT), (HTHH), (TTTT). This gives a total of 16 outcomes.

(a) The outcomes with two heads and two tails are (HHTT), (TTHH), (THTH), (HTHT), (THHT), (HTTH). This gives 6 outcomes.

Therefore, Pr. (getting two heads and two tails) = $\frac{\text{Number of outcomes with two heads and two tails}}{\text{Total number of outcomes}}$

$= \frac{6}{16}$

$= \frac{3}{8}$

(b) The outcome with four tails is (TTTT). This gives 1 outcomes.

Therefore, Pr. (getting four tails) = $\frac{1}{16}$

(c) The outcomes with at least three heads are (HHHH), (HHHT), (THHH), (HHTH), (HTHH). This gives 5 outcomes.

Therefore, Pr. (getting at least three heads) = $\frac{\text{Number of outcomes with at least three heads}}{\text{Total number of outcomes}}$

$= \frac{5}{16}$

(d) The outcomes with at least two heads are (HHHH), (HHHT), (HHTT), (THHH), (TTHH), (THTH), (HTHT) (HHTH), (THHT), (HTTH), (HTHH). This gives 11 outcomes.

Therefore, Pr. (getting at least two heads) = $\frac{\text{Number of outcomes with at least two heads}}{\text{Total number of outcomes}}$

$= \frac{11}{16}$

(e) The outcomes with one head are, (HTTT), (TTTH), (TTHT), (THTT), . This gives 4 outcomes.

Therefore, Pr. (getting one head) = $\frac{\text{Number of outcomes with one head}}{\text{Total number of outcomes}}$

$= \frac{4}{16}$

$= \frac{1}{4}$

(5) A coin is tossed five times. Find the probability of getting at least one tail.

Solution

The total number of outcomes will be $2^5 = 32$

The only outcome without a tail is (HHHHH). This is an outcome of 1

Pr. (getting no tail, i.e. all head) = $\frac{1}{32}$

Therefore, Pr. (getting at least one tail) = 1 - Pr. (getting no tail)

$= 1 - \frac{1}{32}$

$= \frac{31}{32}$

Practice Questions

1. A fair coin is tossed. What is the probability of getting:
(a) a tail
(b) a head
(c) a tail or a head

Solution

(a)

(b)

2. A coin is tossed two times. What is the probability of getting:

(a) a tail and then a head

(b) at least a head

(c) two tails

(d) at least a tail

(e) a head on the first toss, and a tail on the second toss.

Solution

(a)

(b)

(c)

(d)

(e)

3. Three coins are tossed. What is the probability of getting:

(a) three heads

(b) at least one tail

(c) a head, a tail and then a head

(d) at least one head

(e) at least two heads

(f) at most two tails

Solution

(a)

(b)

(c)

(d)

(e)

(f)

4. Four coins are tossed together. Find the probability of getting:

(a) at least one head

(b) four heads

(c) at least two heads

(d) at most three tails

(e) two heads

Solution

(a)

(b)

(c)

(d)

(e)

(5) A coin is tossed five times. Find the probability of getting at least one head.

Answers to Chapter 11

1. (a) $\frac{1}{2}$ (b) $\frac{1}{2}$ (c) 1

2. (a) $\frac{1}{4}$ (b) $\frac{3}{4}$ (c) $\frac{1}{4}$ (d) $\frac{3}{4}$ (e) $\frac{1}{4}$

3. (a) $\frac{1}{8}$ (b) $\frac{7}{8}$ (c) $\frac{1}{8}$ (d) $\frac{7}{8}$ (e) $\frac{1}{2}$ (f) $\frac{7}{8}$

4. (a) $\frac{15}{16}$ (b) $\frac{1}{16}$ (c) $\frac{11}{16}$ (d) $\frac{15}{16}$ (e) $\frac{3}{8}$

5. $\frac{31}{32}$

CHAPTER 12
PROBABILITY ON THROWING OF DICE

Examples

1. A fair die is rolled once. What is the probability of getting:
(a) a number divisible by 3
(b) a multiple of 2
(c) at least 5
(d) at most 2
(e) a prime number or an even number
(f) either a number greater that 2 or a multiple of 4

Solution

(a) Pr. (getting a number divisible by 3) = $\frac{\text{Number of faces having numbers divisible by 3}}{\text{total number of faces}}$

$= \frac{2}{6}$ (Faces with numbers divisible by 3 are 3 and 6, i.e. 2 faces)

$= \frac{1}{3}$

(b) Pr. (getting a multiple of 2) = $\frac{\text{Number of faces having numbers that are multiple of 2}}{\text{total number of faces}}$

$= \frac{3}{6}$ (Faces with numbers that are multiple of 2 are 2, 4 and 6, i.e. 3 faces)

$= \frac{1}{2}$

(c) Pr. (getting at least 5) = $\frac{\text{Number of faces having numbers that are at least 5}}{\text{Total number of faces}}$

$= \frac{2}{6}$ (Faces with numbers that are at least 5 are 5 and 6, i.e. 2 faces)

$= \frac{1}{3}$

(d) Pr. (getting at most 2) = $\frac{\text{Number of faces having numbers that are at least 2}}{\text{Total number of faces}}$

$= \frac{2}{6}$ (Faces with numbers that are at most 2 are 1 and 2, i.e. 2 faces)

$= \frac{1}{3}$

(e) Pr. (getting a prime number or an even number) = $\frac{\text{Number of faces having prime numbers and even numbers}}{\text{Total number of faces}}$

$= \frac{5}{6}$ (Faces with prime numbers are 2, 3, and 5. Faces with even numbers are 2, 4, 6. This will give a total of 5 faces because 2 which is both a prime and even number should be counted once)

Therefore, Pr. (getting a prime number or an even number) = $\frac{5}{6}$

(f) Pr. (getting either a number greater that 2 or a multiple of 4) = $\frac{\text{Number of faces having numb ers greater than 2 and numbers that are multiple of 4}}{\text{Total number of faces}}$

$= \frac{4}{6}$ (Faces with numbers greater than 2 are 3, 4, 5 and 6. Faces with multiple of 4 is 4. This will give a total of 4 faces because 4 which appear in both events should be counted once)

Therefore, Pr. (getting either a number greater that 2 or a multiple of 4) = $\frac{4}{6}$

$= \frac{2}{3}$

2. A die is thrown and a coin is tossed. What is the probability of getting:
(a) a 3 and a head
(b) a tail and a prime number

Solution

(a) From the die, Pr. (getting a 3) = $\frac{1}{6}$

From the coin, Pr. (getting a head) = $\frac{1}{2}$

Since AND means multiplication in probability:

Therefore, Pr. (getting a 3 and a head) = Pr. (getting a 3) x Pr. (getting a head)

$= \frac{1}{6} \times \frac{1}{2}$

$$= \frac{1}{12}$$

(b) (a) From the coin, Pr. (getting a tail) = $\frac{1}{2}$

From the die, Pr. (getting a prime number) = $\frac{3}{6}$ (The prime numbers are 3, i.e. 2, 3 and 5)

$$= \frac{1}{2}$$

Therefore, Pr. (getting a tail and a prime number) = Pr. (getting a tail) x Pr. (getting a prime number)

$$= \frac{1}{2} \times \frac{1}{2}$$

$$= \frac{1}{4}$$

3. Two fair dice are thrown at the same time. Find the probability of getting:
(a) at least one six
(b) a sum of at least 10
(c) a sum of at most 5
(d) a sum less than 3
(e) a total of seven
(f) a sum that is either a prime number or a multiple of 3
(g) a sum that is either divisible by 3 or a multiple of 2

Solution

The outcome table is as shown below. The numbers in the bracket give the outcome from the first and second die respectively. Adding the numbers in the bracket will give the respective sum that will be obtained.

	Number on second die						
	+	1	2	3	4	5	6
	1	(1,1)	(1,2)	(1,3)	(1,4)	(1,5)	(1,6)
Number on	2	(2,1)	(2,2)	(2,3)	(2,4)	(2,5)	(2,6)
first die	3	(3,1)	(3,2)	(3,3)	(3,4)	(3,5)	(3,6)

4	(4,1)	(4,2)	(4,3)	(4,4)	(4,5)	(4,6)
5	(5,1)	(5,2)	(5,3)	(5,4)	(5,5)	(5,6)
6	(6,1)	(6,2)	(6,3)	(6,4)	(6,5)	(6,6)

The outcome table above can be presented in a more direct form by adding the values in the brackets above to obtain the sum. This is as shown below. In the table below, the numbers in the brackets represent the numbers on each die. The numbers that are not in bracket are the outcomes from the sum of numbers on first and second dice.

Number on second die

	+	(1)	(2)	(3)	(4)	(5)	(6)
	(1)	2	3	4	5	6	7
Number on	(2)	3	4	5	6	7	8
first die	(3)	4	5	6	7	8	9
	(4)	5	6	7	8	9	10
	(5)	6	7	8	9	10	11
	(6)	7	8	9	10	11	12

Note that any of the tables above can be used to answer the questions asked above.

(a) The outcomes that can be obtained from getting at least a six are (6,1), (6,2), (6,3), (6,4), (6,5), (6,6), (1,6), (2,6), (3,6), (4,6), (5,6). They are from the first table. They are the outcomes from the 6 on the first die, and 6 on the second die respectively. The number of brackets from this outcome is 11 (when the brackets are counted). Note that the total outcomes from any of the two outcome tables above is 36. This is easier obtained from the second table by counting the numbers that are not in bracket.

Therefore, Pr. (getting at least a six) = $\frac{\text{Number of outcomes obtained when at least a six shows}}{\text{Total number of outcomes on the table}}$

$$= \frac{11}{36}$$

(b) A sum of at least 10 as shown on the second table above are, 10, 10, 10, 11, 11, and 12. This gives a total of 6 outcomes.

Therefore, Pr. (getting a sum of at least 10) = $\frac{6}{36}$ (Note that 36 is the total outcome)

$= \frac{1}{6}$

(c) A sum of at most 5 as shown on the second table above are, 5, 5, 5, 5, 4, 4, 4, 3, 3, and 2. This gives a total of 10 outcomes.

Therefore, Pr. (getting a sum of at most 5) = $\frac{10}{36}$

$= \frac{5}{18}$

(d) A sum less than 3 as shown on the second table above 2 only. This gives a total of 1 outcome.

Therefore, Pr. (getting a sum less than 3) = $\frac{1}{36}$

(e) A total of 7 as shown on the second table above appears 6 times. This gives a total of 6 outcomes.

Therefore, Pr. (getting a total of 7) = $\frac{6}{36}$

$= \frac{1}{6}$

(f) Sums which are prime numbers are 2, 3, 5, 7 and 11. Sums which are multiple of 3 are 3, 6, 9 and 12. Hence we are to count the outcomes from 2, 3, 5, 6, 7, 9, 11, and 12 (3 should be counted once). Hence, from the table, 2 appears 1 time, 3 appears 2 times, 5 appears 4 times, 6 appears 5 times, 7 appears 6 times, 9 appears 4 times, 11 appears 2 times, 12 appears 1 time. This gives a total outcome of 1 time + 2 times + 4 times + 5 times + 6 times + 4 times + 2 times + 1 time = 25. This is easier done on the table by counting all 2, 3, 5, 6, 7, 9, 11 and 12. It will also give a total of 25 outcomes.

Therefore, Pr. (getting a sum that is either a prime number or a multiple of 3) = $\frac{25}{36}$

(g) Sums which are divisible by 3 are 3, 6, 9 and 12. Sums which are multiples of 2 are 2, 4, 6, 8, 10 and 12. Hence we are to count the outcomes from 2, 3, 4, 6, 8, 9, 10 and 12 (6 and 12 which appear in both events should be counted once each). Hence, we go to the second table above and count all 2, 3, 4, 6, 8, 9, 10 and 12. It will give a total of 24 outcomes.

Therefore, Pr. (getting a sum that is either divisible by 3 or a multiple of 2) = $\frac{24}{36}$

$= \frac{2}{3}$

4. An unbiased die with faces numbered 1 to 6 is rolled twice. Find the probability that the product of the numbers obtained is:
(a) odd
(b) even
(c) 12
(d) prime
(e) either odd or a multiple of 5

Solution
The outcome table is as shown below. The numbers in brackets are the numbers on the die.

Number on second die

	x	(1)	(2)	(3)	(4)	(5)	(6)
	(1)	1	2	3	4	5	6
Number on	(2)	2	4	6	8	10	12
first die	(3)	3	6	9	12	15	18
	(4)	4	8	12	16	20	24
	(5)	5	10	15	20	25	30
	(6)	6	12	18	24	30	36

(a) All the odd numbers from the outcome table above are 1, 3, 3, 5, 5, 9, 15, 15, 25. This gives a total of 9 outcomes.

Therefore, Pr. (product of numbers is odd) = $\frac{9}{36}$ (Note that the total outcomes is 36)

$= \frac{1}{4}$

(b) Pr. (product of numbers is even) = 1 - Pr. (product of numbers is odd)

$= 1 - \frac{1}{4}$

$$= \frac{3}{4}$$

This can also be obtained by counting all the outcomes that are even numbers in the table above. Total even numbers is 27.

Hence, Pr. (product of numbers is even) = $\frac{27}{36}$

$$= \frac{3}{4} \quad \text{(As obtained before)}$$

(c) Pr. (product of numbers is 12) = $\frac{4}{36}$ (12 appears 4 times in the table)

$$= \frac{1}{9}$$

(d) All the prime numbers are, 2, 2, 3, 3, 5, 5. This gives a total outcomes of 6.

Therefore, Pr. (product of numbers is prime) = $\frac{6}{36}$

$$= \frac{1}{6}$$

(e) All products that are odd numbers are, 1, 3, 3, 5, 5, 9, 15, 15, 25. All products that are multiples of 5 are, 5, 5, 10, 10, 15, 15, 20, 20, 25, 30, 30.

They will both give a total outcome of 15. Note that, 5, 5, 15, 15, 25 are counted once under odd number. They should not be counted under multiples of 5, as this will result to double counting. Hence with this total outcome of 15,

Pr. (product of numbers is either odd or a multiple of 5) = $\frac{15}{36}$

$$= \frac{5}{12}$$

5. Three dice are thrown together. What is the probability of getting a total score of 10?

Solution.

If a die is thrown once, the total outcome is given by $6^1 = 6$. If two dice are thrown, the total outcome is $6^2 = 36$. Similarly, if three dice are thrown, the total outcome will be $6^3 = 216$.

Now, for us to draw a table with 216 outcomes will be very tedious. So, a direct way of solving this problem will be to select the outcomes from each die that will result in a total score of 10. These outcomes are:

(6, 3, 1), (6, 2, 2), (5, 4, 1), (5, 3, 2), (4, 4, 2), (4, 3, 3)

Each of the brackets above can give us 6 outcomes. For example, the first bracket above can give us the following 6 outcomes:

(6, 3, 1): which means - First die shows 6, second die shows 3, third die shows 1

(6, 1, 3): which means - First die shows 6, second die shows 1, third die shows 3

(1, 6, 3): which means - First die shows 1, second die shows 6, third die shows 3

(1, 3, 6): which means - First die shows 1, second die shows 3, third die shows 6

(3, 1, 6): which means - First die shows 3, second die shows 1, third die shows 6

(3, 6, 1): which means - First die shows 3, second die shows 6, third die shows 1

Similarly, each of the other brackets can give us 6 outcomes.

Let us write out our outcome brackets again. They are, (6, 3, 1), (6, 2, 2), (5, 4, 1), (5, 3, 2), (4, 4, 2), (4, 3, 3)

When each of these brackets give us 6 outcomes, then we will obtain a total of 36 (i.e. 6 x 6) outcomes. Recall that our overall outcome table will give us a total of 216 (i.e. 6^3) outcomes.

Therefore, Pr. (getting a total score of 10) = $\frac{36}{216}$

$= \frac{1}{6}$

Practice Questions

1. A fair die is thrown once. Find the probability of getting:
(a) a 5
(b) a 1
(c) a 9
(d) a 2 or 3 or 6

(e) a number less than 6
(f) a prime or an even number

Solution

(a)

(b)

(c)

(d)

2. A fair die is rolled once. What is the probability of getting:
(a) a number divisible by 2
(b) a multiple of 3
(c) at least 2
(d) at most 3
(e) a perfect square or an odd number
(f) either a number greater that 5 or a multiple of 3

Solution

(a)

(b)

(c)

(d)

(e)

(f)

3. A die is thrown and a coin is tossed. What is the probability of getting:
(a) a 5 and a head
(b) a tail and a perfect cube

Solution

(a)

(b)

4. Two fair dice are thrown at the same time. Find the probability of getting:
(a) at least one four
(b) a sum of at least 6
(c) a sum of at most 10
(d) a sum less than 8
(e) a total of 12

(f) a sum that is either a perfect square or a multiple of 5
(g) a sum that is either divisible by 6 or a multiple of 4

Solution

(a)

(b)

(c)

(d)

(e)

(f)

(g)

5. An unbiased die with faces numbered 1 to 6 is rolled twice. Find the probability that the product of the numbers obtained is:

(a) prime

(b) divisible by 6

(c) 9

(d) a factor of 10

(e) either perfect cube or a multiple of 8

Solution

(a)

(b)

(c)

(d)

(e)

(d)

(e)

6. Three dice are thrown together. What is the probability of getting a total score of 11?

Answers to Chapter 12

1. (a) $\frac{1}{6}$ (b) $\frac{1}{6}$ (c) $\frac{1}{6}$ (d) $\frac{1}{2}$ (e) $\frac{5}{6}$ (f) $\frac{5}{6}$

2. (a) $\frac{1}{2}$ (b) $\frac{1}{2}$ (c) $\frac{5}{6}$ (d) $\frac{1}{2}$ (e) $\frac{2}{3}$ (f) $\frac{1}{3}$

3. (a) $\frac{1}{12}$ (b) $\frac{1}{12}$

4. (a) $\frac{11}{36}$ (b) $\frac{13}{18}$ (c) $\frac{11}{12}$ (d) $\frac{7}{12}$ (e) $\frac{1}{36}$ (f) $\frac{7}{18}$ (g) $\frac{7}{18}$

5. (a) $\frac{1}{6}$ (b) $\frac{5}{12}$ (c) $\frac{1}{36}$ (d) $\frac{1}{6}$ (e) $\frac{1}{6}$

6. $\frac{1}{6}$

CHAPTER 13
MISCELLANEOUS PROBLEMS ON PROBABILITY

Examples

1. A box contains two green balls, three yellow balls and four white balls. A ball is picked at random from the box. What is the probability that it is:

(a) green

(b) yellow

(c) white

(d) blue

(e) not white

(f) either yellow or green

Solution

Total number of balls in the box = 2 + 3 + 4 = 9

(a) Pr. (that it is green) = $\frac{\text{Number of green balls}}{\text{Total number of balls in the box}}$

$= \frac{2}{9}$

(b) Pr. (that it is yellow) = $\frac{\text{Number of yellow balls}}{\text{Total number of balls in the box}}$

$= \frac{3}{9}$

$= \frac{1}{3}$

(c) Pr. (that it is white) = $\frac{\text{Number of white balls}}{\text{Total number of balls in the box}}$

$= \frac{4}{9}$

(d) There is no blue ball in the box.

Therefore, Pr. (that it is blue) = 0

(e) Pr. (that it is not white) = 1 - Pr. (that it is white)

$$= 1 - \frac{4}{9}$$

$$= \frac{5}{9}$$

(f) Pr. (that it is either yellow or green) = $\frac{\text{Number of yellow and green balls}}{\text{Total number of balls in the box}}$

$$= \frac{3 + 2}{9}$$

$$= \frac{5}{9}$$

Or,

Pr. (that it is either yellow or green) = Pr. (that it is yellow) + Pr. (that it is green) (Since OR means addition)

$$= \frac{1}{3} + \frac{2}{9}$$

$$= \frac{3 + 2}{9}$$

$$= \frac{5}{9} \quad \text{(As obtained before)}$$

2. A letter is chosen at random from the word COMPUTER. What is the probability that it is:
(a) either in the word MORE or in the word CUT
(b) either in the word COPE or in the word CUTE
(c) neither in the word ROT nor in the word CUP

Solution
(a) The total number of letters in COMPUTER is 8 letters.

In the word MORE, the number of letters is 4, while in the word CUT, the number of letters is 3. They both give a total of 7 letters.

Therefore, Pr. (that it is either in the word MORE or in the word CUT) = $\frac{7}{8}$

(b) In the word COPE, the number of letters is 4, while in the word CUTE, the number of letters is 4. Without counting any letter twice (i.e. C and E), the two words give a total of 6 letters (i.e. C, O, P, E, U, T).

Therefore, Pr. (that it is either in the word COPE or in the word CUTE) = $\frac{6}{8}$ (The total number of letters in COMPUTER is 8 letters).

$= \frac{3}{4}$

(c) Out of the 8 letters in COMPUTER, the letters that are neither in the word ROT nor in the word CUP are letters M and E. They are 2 letters.

Therefore, Pr. (that it is neither in the word ROT nor in the word CUP) = $\frac{2}{8}$

$= \frac{1}{4}$

(3) In a college 80% of the boys and 45% of the girls can drive a car. If a boy and a girl are chosen at random, what is the probability that:
(a) both of then can drive a car |
(b) the boy cannot drive a car and the girl can drive a car
(c) neither of them can drive a car?
(d) one of them can drive a car

Solution
The probabilities are given in percentage. Hence the total for each probability is 100%

Therefore, Pr. (a boy can drive a car) = $\frac{80}{100}$

$= \frac{4}{5}$

Pr. (a boy cannot drive a car) = $\frac{20}{100}$ (i.e. 100 - 80 = 20)

$= \frac{1}{5}$ (Can also be obtained from $1 - \frac{4}{5}$)

Similarly, Pr. (a girl can drive a car) = $\frac{45}{100}$

$= \frac{9}{20}$ (After equal division by 5)

Pr. (a girl cannot drive a car) = $1 - \frac{9}{20})$

$= \frac{11}{20}$

(a) Therefore, Pr. (both of them can drive a car) = Pr. (a boy can drive a car) AND Pr. (a girl can drive a car)

= Pr. (a boy can drive a car) x Pr. (a girl can drive a car)

$= \frac{4}{5} \text{ X } \frac{9}{20}$

$= \frac{36}{100}$

$= \frac{9}{25}$

(b) Pr. (the boy cannot drive a car and the girl can drive a car) = Pr. (a boy cannot drive a car) AND Pr. (a girl can drive a car)

= Pr. (a boy cannot drive a car) x Pr. (a girl can drive a car)

$= \frac{1}{5} \text{ X } \frac{9}{20}$

$= \frac{9}{100}$

(c) Pr. (neither of them can drive a car) = Pr. (a boy cannot drive a car) AND Pr. (a girl cannot drive a car)

= Pr. (a boy cannot drive a car) x Pr. (a girl cannot drive a car)

$= \frac{1}{5} \text{ X } \frac{11}{20}$

$= \frac{11}{100}$

(d) Since we do not know which of then can drive a car, then this case is logically explained as follows:

Pr. (one of them can drive a car) = either the boy can drive a car AND the girl cannot drive a car OR the girl can drive a car AND the boy cannot drive a car.

This in now calculated as follows:

Pr. (one of them can drive a car) = Pr. (the boy can drive a car) x Pr. (the girl cannot drive a car) + Pr. (the girl can drive a car) x Pr. (the boy cannot drive a car)

$$= (\frac{4}{5} \times \frac{11}{20}) + (\frac{9}{20} \times \frac{1}{5})$$

$$= \frac{11}{25} + \frac{9}{100}$$

$$= \frac{44 + 9}{100}$$

$$= \frac{53}{100}$$

4. The probability of a seed germinating is $\frac{2}{5}$. If three of the seeds are planted, what is the probability that:

(a) none will germinate
(b) at least one will germinate
(c) at least one will not germinate
(d) only one will germinate

Solution

This is a case of selection of three items from two possible events. We are going to write our outcomes in bracket like a tree diagram method. In order to write out the outcomes, let us use the letter G to represent germinate and letter N to represent not germinate.

Hence the outcomes are written as follows:

(GGG), (GGN), (GNG), (GNN), (NGG), (NGN), (NNG), (NNN)

(a) The probability that none will germinate is given by (NNN).

From the question, the probability that a seed germinate, G = $\frac{2}{5}$. Therefore the probability that it will not germinate, N = 1 - G = 1 - $\frac{2}{5} = \frac{3}{5}$

Hence, G = $\frac{2}{5}$, N = $\frac{3}{5}$

Therefore, Pr. (that none will germinate) = (NNN)

$$= \frac{3}{5} \times \frac{3}{5} \times \frac{3}{5}$$

$$= \frac{27}{125}$$

(b) The outcomes of the probability that at least one will germinate are, (GGG), (GGN), (GNG), (GNN), (NGG), (NGN), (NNG). Hence we can compute each of the outcomes and add them together. But this will be tedious. An easier way of solving this problem is as explained below.

The difference between the outcome in question (a) and (b) is (NNN). This shows that subtracting (NNN) from the total probability will give us the outcomes in question (b). Recall that the total of any probability is 1. Therefore, 1 - (NNN) = outcomes in (b)

Hence, Pr. (that at least one will germinate) = 1 - (NNN)

$= 1 - \frac{27}{125}$ [Note that (NNN) = $\frac{27}{125}$ as calculated in question (a)]

$$= \frac{108}{125}$$

(c) The outcomes of the probability that at least one will not germinate are, (GGN), (GNG), (GNN), (NGG), (NGN), (NNG), (NNN). Similar to (b) above, the difference between this outcomes of this question and the overall outcomes is (GGG).

Therefore, Pr. (that at least one will not germinate) = 1 - (GGG)

Let us calculate (GGG) as follows:

Pr. [that all three will germinate, i.e. (GGG)] $= \frac{2}{5} \times \frac{2}{5} \times \frac{2}{5}$

$$= \frac{8}{125}$$

Therefore, Pr. (that at least one will not germinate) = 1 - (GGG)

$$= 1 - \frac{8}{125}$$

$$= \frac{117}{125}$$

(d) The outcomes of the probability that only one will germinate are, (GNN), (NGN), (NNG). Hence we will calculate each of these outcomes and add them together.

(GNN) = Pr. (that the first will germinate) x Pr. (that the second will not germinate) x Pr. (that the third will not germinate)

$$= \frac{2}{5} \times \frac{3}{5} \times \frac{3}{5}$$

$$= \frac{18}{125}$$

$$(NGN) = \frac{3}{5} \times \frac{2}{5} \times \frac{3}{5}$$

$$= \frac{18}{125}$$

$$(NNG) = \frac{3}{5} \times \frac{3}{5} \times \frac{2}{5}$$

$$= \frac{18}{125}$$

Therefore, Pr. (that only one will germinate) $= \frac{18}{125} + \frac{18}{125} + \frac{18}{125}$

$$= \frac{54}{125}$$

5. When children are born, they are equally likely to be boys or girls. What is the probability that in a family of four children:

(a) three are boys and one is a girl

(b) at least two are girls

(c) two are boys and two are girls

(d) the first and second born are girls

Solution

Since children are equally likely to be boys or girls, it means that the probability of having a boy is $\frac{1}{2}$, and the probability of having a girl is also $\frac{1}{2}$. This is similar to the case of tossing a coin (i.e. $\frac{1}{2}$ for head and $\frac{1}{2}$ for tail).

Therefore, the case of a family of four children is like when four coins are tossed. Refer to the example on tossing four coins in chapter 4.

Let us use B for boy and G for girl to write out the total outcomes of 16 (i.e. $2^4 = 16$) as shown below.

The outcomes are: (BBBB), (BBBG), (BBGG), (BGGG), (GBBB), (GGBB), (GGGB), (GBGB), (BGBG), (BBGB), (GBBG), (BGGB), (GGBG), (GBGG), (BGBB), (GGGG). This gives a total of 16 outcomes.

(a) The outcomes that the children are three boys and one girl are, (BBBG), (GBBB), (BBGB), (BGBB). This gives 4 outcomes.

Therefore, Pr. (three are boys and one is a girl) = $\frac{4}{16}$

$= \frac{1}{4}$

(b) The outcomes that the children are at least two girls are, (BBGG), (BGGG), (GGBB), (GGGB), (GBGB), (BGBG), (GBBG), (BGGB), (GGBG), (GBGG), (GGGG). This gives 11 outcomes.

Therefore, Pr. (at least two are girls) = $\frac{11}{16}$

(c) The outcomes that the children are two boys and two girls are, (BBGG), (GGBB), (GBGB), (BGBG), (GBBG), (BGGB). This gives 6 outcomes.

Therefore, Pr. (two are boys and two are girls) = $\frac{6}{16}$

$= \frac{3}{8}$

(d) The outcomes that the first and second born are girls are, (GGBB), (GGGB), (GGBG), (GGGG). This gives 4 outcomes.

Therefore, Pr. (the first and second born are girls) = $\frac{4}{16}$

$= \frac{1}{4}$

6. A bag contains three blue balls, four red balls and five white balls. Three balls are removed from the bag without replacement. What is the probability of getting:
(a) a white, blue and red balls in that order
(a) one of each colour
(c) at least two white balls

Solution

The total number of balls in the bag = 3 + 4 + 5 = 12

(a) A white, blue and red balls in that order means that the first is white, the second is blue and the third is red. This can be represented as (WBR).

Note that this is a case of without replacement. Hence after each ball is removed, the total number of ball remaining and the number of the particular ball removed are both reduced by one.

Therefore, Pr. (getting a white, blue and red balls, i.e. WBR) = $\frac{5}{12} \times \frac{3}{11} \times \frac{4}{10}$. (Notice how the total balls is reduced by 1 after each ball is removed from the bag.

$$= \frac{60}{1320}$$

$$= \frac{1}{22} \qquad \text{(After equal division by 60)}$$

(b) Let B represent blue, R represent red and W represent white. Then the outcomes for getting one of each colour are given by: (BRW), (BWR), (RBW), (RWB), (WBR), (WRB).

Let us now calculate each of them.

(BRW) = Pr. (First is blue) x Pr. (Second is red) x Pr. (Third is white)

$$= \frac{3}{12} \times \frac{4}{11} \times \frac{5}{10}$$

$$= \frac{1}{4} \times \frac{4}{11} \times \frac{1}{2}$$

$$= \frac{4}{88}$$

$$= \frac{1}{22}$$

Similarly, each of the other five outcomes, i.e. (BWR), (RBW), (RWB), (WBR), (WRB), will each give us a value of $\frac{1}{22}$ when calculated. This is because each is obtained by multiplying 3 x 4 x 5, to give the numerator, and 12 x 11 x 10, to give the denominator, which simplifies to $\frac{1}{22}$.

Therefore, Pr. (getting one of each colour) = $\frac{1}{22} + \frac{1}{22} + \frac{1}{22} + \frac{1}{22} + \frac{1}{22} + \frac{1}{22}$

$$= \frac{6}{22}$$

$$= \frac{3}{11}$$

(c) Let us write out a different outcome for this problem. Since we are concerned about one colour, we are going to use W to represent white colour, and N to represent not a white colour. This will give us 8 outcomes in brackets as usual. The outcomes are:

(WWW), (WWN), (WNW), (WNN), (NWW), (NWN), (NNW), (NNN).

The outcomes representing at least two white balls are: (WWW), (WWN), (WNW), (NWW).

Number of white balls is 5. Therefore number of balls that are not white = 12 - 5 = 7, or blue + red = 3 + 4 = 7. (Blue and red ball are the balls that are not white balls).

Let us now calculate each of the outcomes above as follows:

(WWW) = Pr. (first is white) x Pr. (second is white) x Pr. (third is white)

$= \frac{5}{12} \times \frac{4}{11} \times \frac{3}{10}$ (Take note of the reduction in the white balls and total number of balls as each ball is removed from the bag)

$= \frac{60}{1320}$

$= \frac{1}{22}$

(WWN) $= \frac{5}{12} \times \frac{4}{11} \times \frac{7}{10}$ (Note that there are 7 balls that are not white)

$= \frac{140}{1320}$

$= \frac{7}{66}$

(WNW) $= \frac{5}{12} \times \frac{7}{11} \times \frac{4}{10}$

$= \frac{140}{1320}$

$= \frac{7}{66}$

(NWW) $= \frac{7}{12} \times \frac{5}{11} \times \frac{4}{10}$

$= \frac{140}{1320}$

$$= \frac{7}{66}$$

Therefore, Pr. (getting at least two white balls) = (WWW) or (WWN) or (WNW) or (NWW)

= (WWW) + (WWN) + (WNW) + (NWW)

$$= \frac{1}{22} + \frac{7}{66} + \frac{7}{66} + \frac{7}{66}$$

$$= \frac{3 + 7 + 7 + 7}{66}$$

$$= \frac{24}{66}$$

$$= \frac{4}{11}$$

7. A committee consist of 6 men and 4 women. A subcommittee made up of three members is randomly chosen from the committee members. What is the probability that:
(a) they are all men
(b) two of them are women?

Solution

Let us write out the outcome for this problem. Let M represent man, and W represent woman. This will give us 8 outcomes in brackets as usual. The outcomes are:

(WWW), (WWM), (WMW), (WMM), (MWW), (MWM), (MMW), (MMM).

(a) The total members in the committee are: 6 + 4 = 10.

The outcomes representing all men is (MMM)

Therefore, Pr. (they are all men, i.e. MMM) = Pr. (first is a man) x Pr. (second is a man) x Pr. (third is a man)

$= \frac{6}{10} \text{x} \frac{5}{9} \text{x} \frac{4}{8}$ (Notice the reduction in the number of men and people left, as each member is chosen from the committee).

$$= \frac{130}{720}$$

$$= \frac{13}{72}$$

(b) The outcomes showing that two of them are women are: (WWM), (WMW), (MWW)

Let us calculate each of them as follows:

(WWM) = Pr. (the first is a woman) x Pr. (the second is a woman) x Pr. (the third is a man)

$$= \frac{4}{10} \times \frac{3}{9} \times \frac{6}{8}$$

$$= \frac{72}{720}$$

$$= \frac{1}{10}$$

$$(WMW) = \frac{4}{10} \times \frac{6}{9} \times \frac{3}{8}$$

$$= \frac{72}{720}$$

$$= \frac{1}{10}$$

$$(MWW) = \frac{6}{10} \times \frac{4}{9} \times \frac{3}{8}$$

$$= \frac{72}{720}$$

$$= \frac{1}{10}$$

Therefore, Pr. (two of them are women) = (WWM) or (WMW) or (MWW)

= (WWM) + (WMW) + (MWW)

$$= \frac{1}{10} + \frac{1}{10} + \frac{1}{10}$$

$$= \frac{3}{10}$$

8. A box contains seven blue pens and three red pens. Three pens are picked one after the other without replacement. Find the probability of picking:

(a) two blue pens

(b) at least two red pens

(c) at most two blue pens

Solution

Let B represent blue pen, and R represent red pen. The outcomes are:

(BBB), (BBR), (BRB), (BRR), (RBB), (RBR), (RRB), (RRR).

The total number of pens = 7 + 3 = 10

(a) The outcomes showing two blue pens are: (BBR), (BRB), (RBB)

Let us calculate each of them as follows:

(BBR) = Pr. (the first is a blue pen) x Pr. (the second is a blue pen) x Pr. (the third is a red pen)

$$= \frac{7}{10} \times \frac{6}{9} \times \frac{3}{8}$$

$$= \frac{126}{720}$$

$$= \frac{7}{40}$$ (In its lowest term after equal division by 18)

$$(BRB) = \frac{7}{10} \times \frac{3}{9} \times \frac{6}{8}$$

$$= \frac{126}{720}$$

$$= \frac{7}{40}$$

Also, $(RBB) = \frac{7}{40}$ (Similar to the once above)

Therefore, Pr. (picking two blue pens) = $\frac{7}{40} \times \frac{7}{40} \times \frac{7}{40}$

$$= \frac{21}{40}$$

(b) The outcomes representing at least two red pens are: (RRR), (RRB), (RBR), (BRR)

Let us now calculate each of the outcomes as follows:

(RRR) = Pr. (first is a red pen) x Pr. (second is a red pen) x Pr. (third is a red pen)

$= \frac{3}{10} \times \frac{2}{9} \times \frac{1}{8}$ (Take note of the reduction in the red pens and total number of pens as each pen is picked from the box)

$= \frac{6}{720}$

$= \frac{1}{120}$

(RRB) $= \frac{3}{10} \times \frac{2}{9} \times \frac{7}{8}$

$= \frac{42}{720}$

$= \frac{7}{120}$

Hence, (RBR) $= \frac{7}{120}$ (This is similar to the one above)

And, (BRR) $= \frac{7}{120}$ (Same reason as above)

Therefore, Pr. (picking at least two red pens) $= \frac{1}{120} + \frac{7}{120} + \frac{7}{120} + \frac{7}{120}$

$= \frac{1+7+7+7}{120}$

$= \frac{22}{120}$

$= \frac{11}{60}$

(c) The outcomes that represent picking at most two blue pens are: (BBR), (BRB), (BRR), (RBB), (RBR), (RRB), (RRR). Note that at most two blue pens means 2, 1 or 0 blue pens.

Notice that there is only (BBB) missing from this outcome. This shows that it can be obtained by: total probability - (BBB). Which is: 1 - (BBB).

Let us calculate (BBB) as follows:

(BBB) = Pr. (first is a blue pen) x Pr. (second is a blue pen) x Pr. (third is a blue pen)

$= \frac{7}{10} \times \frac{6}{9} \times \frac{5}{8}$

$$= \frac{210}{720}$$

$$= \frac{7}{24}$$ (After equal division by 30)

Therefore, Pr. (picking at most two blue pens) = 1 - (BBB)

$$= 1 - \frac{7}{24}$$

$$= \frac{17}{24}$$

Practice Questions

1. A box contains 5 green balls, 8 yellow balls and 7 white balls. A ball is picked at random from the box. What is the probability that it is:
(a) green
(b) yellow
(c) white
(d) blue
(e) not white
(f) either yellow or green

Solution

(a)

(b)

(c)

(d)

(e)

(f)

2. A letter is chosen at random from the word NORMADIC. What is the probability that it is:
(a) either in the word MAD or in the word CORN
(b) either in the word NORM or in the word DAM
(c) neither in the word RID nor in the word CAN

Solution

(a)

(b)

(c)

(3) In a college 20% of the boys and 8% of the girls who had graduated from the college, graduated with distinction since the inception of the college. If a boy and a girl are chosen at random, what is the probability that:
(a) both of them will graduate with distinction
(b) the boy will not and the girl will graduate with distinction

(c) neither of them will graduate with distinction?
(d) one of them will graduate with distinction

Solution

(a)

(b)

(c)

(d)

4. The probability of a seed germinating is $\frac{1}{4}$. If three of the seeds are planted, what is the probability that:
(a) none will germinate
(b) at least one will germinate
(c) at least one will not germinate
(d) only one will germinate

Solution

(a)

(b)

(c)

(d)

5. When parents who are carriers of sickle cell disorder get married, they are equally likely to give birth to normal child and sick child. What is the probability that in a family of three children:

(a) two are normal and one is sick

(b) at least two are sick

(c) one is normal and two are sick

(d) the first is sick

(e) at most one is normal

Solution

(a)

(b)

(c)

(d)

(e)

6. A box contains six blue balls, three red balls and five white balls. Three balls are removed from the bag without replacement. What is the probability of getting:

(a) a white, blue and red balls in that order

(a) one of each colour

(c) at least two white balls

Solution

(a)

(b)

(c)

7. A committee consist of 4 men and 2 women. A subcommittee made up of two members is randomly chosen from the committee members. What is the probability that:

(a) they are all men

(b) one of them is a woman?

Solution

(a)

(b)

8. A bag contains 5 blue balls and seven red balls. Three balls are picked one after the other without replacement. Find the probability of picking:

(a) two blue balls

(b) at least two red balls

(c) at most two blue balls

Solution

(a)

(b)

(c)

Answers to Chapter 13

1. (a) $\frac{1}{4}$ (b) $\frac{2}{5}$ (c) $\frac{7}{20}$ (d) 0 (e) $\frac{13}{20}$ (f) $\frac{13}{20}$

2. (a) $\frac{7}{8}$ (b) $\frac{3}{4}$ (c) $\frac{1}{4}$

3. (a) $\frac{2}{125}$ (b) $\frac{8}{125}$ (c) $\frac{92}{125}$ (d) $\frac{31}{125}$

4. (a) $\frac{27}{64}$ (b) $\frac{37}{64}$ (c) $\frac{63}{64}$ (d) $\frac{27}{64}$

5. (a) $\frac{3}{8}$ (b) $\frac{1}{2}$ (c) $\frac{3}{8}$ (d) $\frac{1}{2}$ (e) $\frac{1}{2}$

6. (a) $\frac{15}{364}$ (b) $\frac{145}{182}$ (c) $\frac{25}{91}$

7. (a) $\frac{2}{5}$ (b) $\frac{8}{15}$

8. (a) $\frac{7}{22}$ (b) $\frac{7}{11}$ (c) $\frac{21}{22}$

If you have any enquiries, suggestions or information concerning this book, please contact the author through the email below.

KINGSLEY AUGUSTINE

kingzohb2@yahoo.com

Twitter handle: @kingzohb2

www.ingramcontent.com/pod-product-compliance
Lightning Source LLC
Chambersburg PA
CBHW081430220526
45466CB00008B/2330
* 9 7 8 1 6 9 1 5 2 2 1 6 3 *